Interpretation and Uses
of Medical Statistics

GEOFFREY J. BOURKE

M.A., M.D., F.F.C.M., D.P.H., D.I.H., D.C.H.,

Professor of Social and Preventive Medicine,
University College, Dublin
Consultant in Social Medicine and Epidemiology,
St. Vincent's Hospital, Elm Park, Dublin

AND

JAMES McGILVRAY

M.A., M.LITT.,

Research Professor,
Fraser of Allander Institute, University of Strathclyde

SECOND EDITION

BLACKWELL SCIENTIFIC PUBLICATIONS
OXFORD LONDON EDINBURGH MELBOURNE

© 1969, 1975 Blackwell Scientific Publications
Osney Mead, Oxford
85 Marylebone High Street, London, W1M 3DE
9 Forrest Road, Edinburgh
P.O. Box 9, North Balwyn, Victoria, Australia

ISBN 0 632 00228 X

FIRST PUBLISHED 1969
SECOND EDITION 1975

Distributed in the United States of America by
J. B. Lippincott Company, Philadelphia,
and in Canada by
J. B. Lippincott Company of Canada Ltd., Toronto.

Printed in Great Britain by
WESTERN PRINTING SERVICES LTD
BRISTOL

Contents

Chapter 5

Chapter 6

Chapter 7

Preface

The idea to write a book of this kind was prompted by colleagues who have had no formal training in medical statistics. Textbooks available on statistics more often place emphasis on calculation rather than on interpretation, and this apparently has a discouraging effect on medical people. It is clear that there is a need for a book which will assist those interested in medical statistics to become acquainted with the terms and methods commonly employed in the analysis and presentation of data. The book, then, is not intended as a textbook on statistical method. It is designed to aid graduates and undergraduates to understand the scope, logic, and techniques of approach of statistical method as applied to medicine and allied subjects. It will be of particular value to those who are not actively engaged in research and who would have little knowledge of statistics, but who are anxious to keep abreast of advances in medicine and allied subjects by reading journals. We hope that it will also prove useful as an introductory text to a full course in methods of statistical analysis; while emphasis is placed on interpretation certain basic notions of statistical inference are discussed though in a simplified way.

We are indebted to many people who have been of assistance in the course of writing the text. Our thanks are due to the numerous authors who granted us permission to reproduce statistical data from their publications, and to Mr. L. A. Turner, Publishing Manager of the British Medical Journal, for arranging authors' permission in many cases. We are grateful to the Editors of the various journals for their helpful co-operation. We acknowledge the assistance of Dr. Noel Clarke, and Dr. Joseph Masterson, Department of Pathology, University College, Dublin; Mr. David Lyon, Research Associates, London; and Mr. Keith Wilson-Davis, Economic and Social Research

Institute, Dublin; all of whom provided helpful comment with regard to the text. Finally, our thanks are due to our wives for their help and encouragement.

Geoffrey J. Bourke
James McGilvray

January, 1969.

Preface to Second Edition

We are pleased to write a second edition of this book and are grateful to those who by writing to us directly, or who in reviews of the first edition, suggested changes and offered criticism. We have endeavoured to meet relevant criticism in this new edition, and to make appropriate changes.

We owe a debt of gratitude to many people in the preparation of this new edition but we would like especially to thank Professor D. J. Newell of the University, Newcastle-upon-Tyne and Professor Peter Froggatt of The Queen's University of Belfast who wrote to us directly and offered helpful criticism. We hope we have responded in a constructive manner to their efforts.

Some new examples of data have been included in the text and we are indebted to the authors and editors of journals for permission to reproduce these data. A reading list has also been included.

Geoffrey J. Bourke
James McGilvray

April, 1975.

1

1.1 Introduction

A first step in the description and analysis of statistical data is usually to present the data in the form of a table, graph or diagram. This is a convenient way of summarizing the statistics, and also serves to demonstrate to the reader the principal characteristics of the data. In effect, it presents the reader with a compact view of what would otherwise be a jumbled mass of statistics. The exact form in which the data are presented will naturally depend upon the subject matter, as well as upon the methods and aims of the statistical analysis. Most readers will already be familiar with the use of tables and diagrams for these purposes. It is not intended here to give a detailed account of the numerous ways in which data can be presented but by means of examples some general types and features of tables and diagrams will be explained. Emphasis is placed on interpretation rather than construction. In addition, there are certain special types of tables and diagrams used in statistical analysis which are important in relation to subsequent chapters and which will be discussed in greater detail.

While tabular and graphical presentation represents the initial and elementary stages of statistical analysis they are nevertheless extremely important. The way in which statistics are presented is closely related to the aims and techniques of statistical analysis. There is, therefore, a strong interpretative element in the appearance of many tables and graphs. For example, by selecting different scales for a graph quite different impressions can be created.

A fault which is fairly common, is to attempt to show too much in a table or diagram. In general a table or diagram should be self-explanatory without the need for over-elaborate explanatory

1

'keys' or notes. Examples have often been seen in which it is more difficult to interpret a graph than to read the accompanying text. This defeats the purpose of graphical presentation.

1.2 Tabular presentation

The object of a table is to organize and present data in a compact and readily comprehensible form. Some fairly simple tables are illustrated in Examples 1.1–1.5.

In each of these examples the tables are self-explanatory and where necessary units of measurement are specified. The data have been grouped and classified according to some characteristic or characteristics. In Example 1.1 the basis of classification is qualitative, that is by source of referrral. In such a case the characteristic which forms the basis of the classification is referred to as an *attribute*. The figures which appear in the body of the table are referred to as the *frequencies*, and record the total number of observations in each group or class; the sum of the frequencies in each column makes up the *total frequency* or the *total number of observations*.

In Example 1.1 it will be seen that the percentage frequencies are also shown. *Percentage* or *relative* frequencies are quite often used in tables and are useful for comparative purposes. In the example quoted the percentage distributions facilitate a comparison of source of referral between males and females.

In Examples 1.2 and 1.3 the characteristic which forms the basis of the classification is quantitative or numerical, and is referred to as a *variable*.* Thus, in Example 1.2, age is the variable and in Example 1.3 the variable is the number of admissions to hospital. Both tables are examples of what is called a *frequency distribution*. The two distributions, however, differ in one impor-

---

* Sometimes a number is used to represent what is essentially an attribute. If the population of a city is classified according to electoral ward and each ward identified by number rather than by name then the basis of the classification will be numerical. However, the characteristic selected (ward number) cannot be regarded as a variable in the sense in which it is used here. The numerical unit is not a unit of measurement but merely a tag or label.

tant respect. In Example 1.2 the variable is *continuous*, and in Example 1.3 the variable is *discrete*. A discrete variable is one which varies by finite specific steps. In Example 1.3 the variable takes integral values only; numbers such as $1\cdot4$ or $3\frac{1}{2}$ cannot be used. In Example 1.2 the variable is continuous and can therefore take any value. A continuous variable is one which given any two values, however close together, an intermediate value can always be found. Examples of continuous variables are time, temperature, and age, while examples of discrete variables are number of children per family, number of hospital admissions, or numbers of tablets in bottles of different sizes.

In practice variables which are continuous are measured in discrete units and age (Example 1.2) may be measured to the nearest year or in other instances to the nearest month. It is important, however, to understand the difference between continuous and discrete variables.

In Example 1.2 the data have been grouped into thirteen different classes. The first class is 10–14, the second is 15–19 and so on. The difference between the *lower class limit* and the *upper class limit* of each class is called the *class interval*. The lower class limit of the initial class in Example 1.2 is 10. However, since age is a continuous variable values such as $10\cdot2$ and $10\cdot7$ are permissible, and the lower class limit may be written $10\cdot0$. The upper class limit may appear to be 14. However, a value of $14\cdot9$ or $14\cdot99$ would be included in the first class and the true upper class limit is in fact $14\cdot999\ldots$. Thus, the class interval is $14\cdot999\ldots$ *minus* $10\cdot0 = 4\cdot999\ldots$ or, more conveniently, $5\cdot0$ years. This class then could have been designated '10 years and under 15 years'. In Example 1.2 the class interval for each class is 5 years and the distribution has equal class intervals.

Another important concept is the *class mid-point* the use of which will be referred to in the next chapter. This is the value of the variable mid-way between the lower class limit and upper class limit. The class mid-point for the first class in Example 1.2 is $12\cdot5$, the mid-point of the second class is $17\cdot5$, and so on.

The notions of class intervals and class mid-points cannot be

EXAMPLE 1.1

Distribution of patients in hospital by source of referral

Source of Referral	Male	%	Female	%	Total	%
Other hospital	64	6·9	33	3·4	97	5·1
General practitioner	346	37·5	423	43·1	769	40·3
Out-patient department	273	29·5	350	35·6	623	32·7
Casualty	161	17·4	95	9·7	256	13·4
Other (including unknown)	80	8·7	81	8·2	161	8·5
Total	924	100·0	982	100·0	1,906	100·0

Reprinted from the *Dublin General Hospital and Geriatric Study*.
Bourke G. J., and Coughlan J. A. (1966), p. 8. (Table abbreviated.)
(By permission of the Authors and the Medical Research Council
of Ireland.)

EXAMPLE 1.2

Age distribution of 1,773 male Assam labour force

Age (years)	No.
10–14	30
15–19	160
20–24	182
25–29	279
30–34	254
35–39	248
40–44	197
45–49	161
50–54	121
55–59	74
60–64	43
65–69	18
70–74	6
Total subjects	1,773

Reprinted from the *British Journal of Preventive and Social
Medicine*. Wilson J. M. G. (1958), **12**, 204. Arterial blood pressure
in plantation workers in North-East India. (Table abbreviated.)
(By permission of the Author, Editor, and Publishers.)

EXAMPLE 1.3

Frequency of admission to hospital of patients aged 65 years and over (fit and remediable)

No. of admissions to hospital past 5 years	Male	%	Female	%	Total	%
1	40	44·9	49	49·0	89	47·1
2	12	13·6	27	27·0	39	20·6
3	19	21·3	11	11·0	30	15·9
4–7	15	16·9	10	10·0	25	13·2
8–11	2	2·2	2	2·0	4	2·1
12–15	1	1·1	1	1·0	2	1·1
15+	0	0·0	0	0·0	0	0·0
Total	89	100·0	100	100·0	189	100·0

Reprinted from the *Dublin General Hospital and Geriatric Study.* Bourke G. J., and Coughlan J. A. (1966), p.29. (Table abbreviated.) (By permission of the Authors and the Medical Research Council of Ireland.)

EXAMPLE 1.4

Number of tracheostomies performed yearly

Year	No. of tracheostomies
1950	8
1951	12
1952	17
1953	18
1954	31
1955	53
1956	49
1957	62
1958	63
1959	76
Total	389

Reprinted from the *British Medical Journal.* McClelland R. M. A. (1965), **2**, 567. Complications of tracheostomy. (Table abbreviated.) (By permission of the Author, Editor, and Publishers.)

EXAMPLE 1.5

Distribution of pesticides in human fat by age and residue level

Pesticide	Residue range (p.p.m.)	Age group in years		
		1–39	40–63	64–88
Total B.H.C.	0·0–0·2	⑨	4	2
	0·3–0·4	7	8	⑨
	0·5–1·0	6	10	⑪
Dieldrin	0·0–0·1	13	3	4
	0·2	9	5	4
	0·3–0·9	0	14	14
Total D.D.T.-equivalent	0·0–1·9	11	2	4
	2·0–3·9	7	12	11
	4·0–8·9	4	⑧	7

Reprinted from the *British Medical Journal*. Egan H., Goulding R., Roburn J., and Tatton J. O'G. (1965), **2**, 66. Organo-chlorine pesticide residues in human fat and human milk. (By permission of the Authors, Editor, and Publishers.)

applied in quite the same way to discrete frequency distributions. Thus in Example 1.3 the values 1, 2, and 3 cannot be interpreted as 1·0 to 1·999..., 2·0 to 2·999..., 3·0 to 3·999.... The variable takes only the integral values 1·0, 2·0, and 3·0, and there are no class intervals. To the extent that higher integral values are grouped together in this table, they may be said to form classes but the class 4–7 cannot be interpreted to mean that the variable can take non-integral values between 4·0 and 8·0.

Example 1.4 illustrates another common type of table. This is a *time series* which records the variation in the value of some variable, in this case number of tracheostomies performed annually, over a period of time.

In Examples 1.1–1.3 the data have been classified or grouped on the basis of a single characteristic (source of referral, age, number of admissions). Example 1.5 illustrates what is called a *bi-variate classification* which as its name suggests is a classification according to two variables. There are in fact three separate bi-variate classifications in this example, the pairs of variables in each case being (a) Total B.H.C. and age, (b) Dieldrin and age, and (c) Total D.D.T.-equivalent and age, respectively. In each case the observations are first arranged in groups according to residue range. In the case of Total B.H.C./Age there are 15 persons in the range 0·0–0·2, 24 in the range 0·3–0·4, and 27 in the range 0·5–1·0. Each group is then further sub-divided according to age. The class into which each observation falls is therefore determined by two characteristics.

Bi-variate classifications of this kind are widely used in statistical analysis and will be further considered in a later chapter.* They are designed principally to show whether or not there is any association between the two variables concerned. In the example quoted inspection of the B.H.C./Age classification appears to suggest some association between age and residue range. The table demonstrates a tendency for those with a low residue range to be in the lower age groups whilst most of the older subjects fall into the higher residue range category.

1.3 Diagrammatic presentation

Graphs and diagrams of various kinds are often a very effective means of presenting data. Some common types of diagrams are shown in the figures and examples which follow.

The first four are similar in appearance and represent various forms of *bar charts*. The attribute or variable is shown on the horizontal axis (abscissa) and the frequency, or relative frequency, is measured on the vertical axis (ordinate). Sometimes, however, the variable is shown on the vertical axis and the frequency on the horizontal. Bars are constructed to show the frequency, or relative frequency, for each class of the attribute or variable. Usually the bars are equal in width, although this is not always the case as will be explained shortly. Figure 1.1 is a simple bar chart illustrating the data relating to males in Example 1.1. The height of the bar shows the frequency of each group and gives a useful 'picture' of the distribution.

---

* Multi-variate classifications, involving more than two variables, are also used although they are more difficult to present in tabular form.

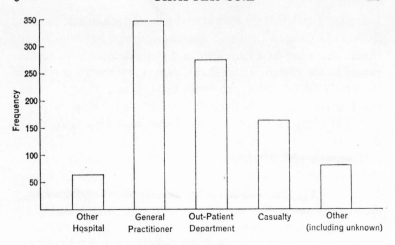

FIG. 1.1 Bar chart of data (males only) in Example 1.1. Distribution of 924 male patients in hospital by source of referral

EXAMPLE 1.6

Multiple bar chart.
Percentage infestation of Asian boys (637 cases)

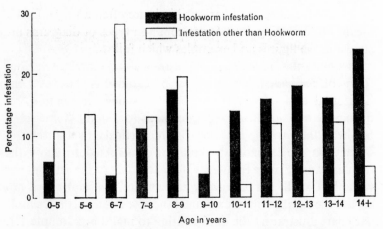

Reprinted from the *British Medical Journal*. Archer D. M., Bamford F. N., and Lees E. (1965), **2**, 1517. Helminth infestations in immigrant children. (By permission of the Authors, Editor, and Publishers.)

EXAMPLE 1.7

Composite bar chart.

Total number of cases, total women, and total women aged 18–45 who were found to have cerebral arterial occlusion in each year from 1955. (The figure for 1965 is for the first six months only.)

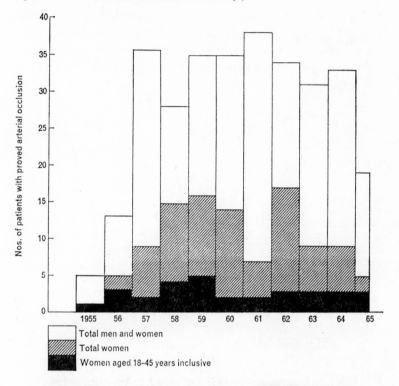

Reprinted from the *British Medical Journal*. Illis L., Kocen R. S., McDonald W. I., and Mondkar V. P. (1965), 2, 1164. Oral contraceptives and cerebral arterial occlusion. (By permission of the Authors, Editor, and Publishers.)

In Example 1.6, two frequency distributions have been super-imposed on the same diagram. By this means a visual comparison can be made between hookworm and other forms of infestation at each age group. Note that each bar measures the *relative frequency* at each age group.

Example 1.7 represents what is called a *composite bar chart*. As before the height of each bar is directly proportional to the frequency but each bar is sub-divided, by shading and hatching, to show the share of different groups in the total frequency. Interest here is not simply in the total number of arterial occlusions but in their distribution amongst men and women, and women of particular ages. In this example it will be noted that the last bar, for 1965, is only half the width of the others. This is because the figures for 1965 relate to the first 6 months only. Bars are drawn equal in width if the frequency distribution has equal class intervals.

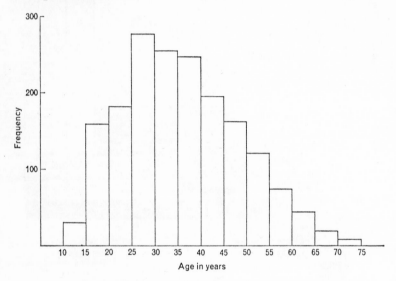

Fɪɢ. 1.2. Histogram of data in Example 1.2. Age distribution of 1,773 male Assam labour force

Figure 1.2 is a special and important type of bar chart called a *histogram*. Since the class intervals in this distribution are equal (5 years) the width of each bar of the histogram is the same and the area of each bar is directly proportional to the frequency of the corresponding class of the frequency distribution. The total area of all the bars is proportional to the total frequency. The histogram gives a good picture of the shape of the distribution showing it to rise to a peak in the 25 and under 30 age group and then to slowly decline thereafter. This histogram is further discussed below.

EXAMPLE 1.8

Time series graph.
Incidence of hookworm and other infestation in Asian children.

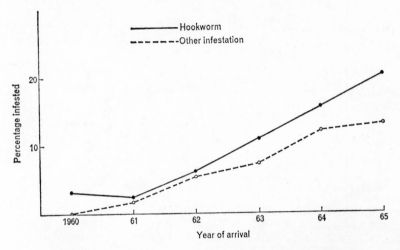

Year of arrival

Reprinted from the *British Medical Journal.* Archer D. M., Bamford F. N., and Lees E. (1965), **2,** 1517. Helminth infestations in immigrant children. (By permission of the Authors, Editor, and Publishers.)

Example 1.8 is a time series *graph.* The percentage infestation detected in 1965 and related to year of arrival is plotted on the graph and represented by a dot. Thus, it can be seen that approximately 3% of Asian children who had immigrated in 1960 had hookworm infestation, whilst 'other' infestation was negligible. The percentage of infestation detected shows an increase for each year since 1961; one explanation for this is that more recent arrivals have had less opportunity for diagnosis and treatment. Frequently, as in this example, the dots or plot points on the graph are joined together to show the 'trend' from year to year. The graph here indicates a fairly constant upward trend.

Example 1.9 represents another important type of diagram, called a *scatter diagram.* Like a bi-variate classification, a scatter

B

EXAMPLE 1.9

Scatter diagram.
Birth-weights in primiparae in Aberdeen.

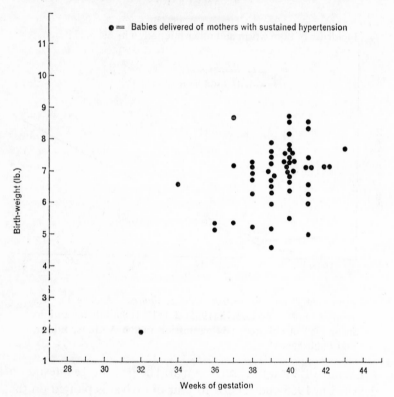

Reprinted from the *Lancet*. Walters W. A. W. (1966), **2**, 1214.
Effects of sustained maternal hypertension on foetal growth and
survival. (Table abbreviated.) (By permission of the Author,
Editor, and Publishers.)

diagram is designed to show the association, or lack of association, between two variables. One variable is measured along each
axis. For each subject, or whatever the unit of observation might
be, a pair of readings is taken in respect of each variable. A point
is then plotted on the graph in relation to the two readings. Thus
in Example 1.9 there will be noticed one extreme point in the

lower left-hand corner of the diagram. This point corresponds to a gestation period of 32 weeks and a birth-weight of just under 2 lb. Other points on the scatter diagram are similarly plotted. Clearly the intention in this particular example is to show the association, if any, between weeks of gestation and birth-weight of babies among mothers with sustained hypertension. One might expect that the longer the gestation period the greater the birth-weight, in which case one would expect the scatter of points to show an upward 'trend' to the right. Inspection of the scatter diagram does not lend strong support to this hypothesis although there *is* a tendency for long gestations to be associated with higher birth-weights. In a later chapter various techniques for measuring associations of this kind will be explained.

Finally, Example 1.10 illustrates a *semi-logarithmic (or ratio) chart*. This is very similar to a scatter diagram except that one of the variables is measured on a logarithmic scale rather than on an arithmetic scale. Sometimes both variables are measured on a logarithmic scale; this is then called a logarithmic chart. In the example shown urinary pH is measured normally on the arithmetic scale. The vertical axis, however, measures the logarithm value of urobilinogen output and it is the logarithm value which is plotted against pH. The right-hand vertical axis, incidentally, shows the arithmetic or natural numbers corresponding to the log value scale. Thus, the natural number corresponding to the logarithm value 1·0 is 10, the natural number 1·0 corresponds to the log value zero and so on. Inspection of the scatter diagram shows that there is a tendency for high values of urinary pH to be associated with high values of urobilinogen output as measured on a logarithmic scale.

Why use a logarithmic scale rather than an arithmetic scale ? To understand this the following property of a logarithmic scale may be noted: Equal vertical distances on a logarithmic scale measure equal *proportionate differences* whereas equal vertical distances on an arithmetic scale measure equal *absolute differences*. Thus, suppose we extended the left-hand axis of Example 1.10 until we reached the logarithm value 2·0 (which would bring the axis up nearly to the top of the page), the difference between log value 1·0

EXAMPLE 1.10

Semi-logarithmic chart.
Urobilinogen output in a normal subject related to urinary pH.

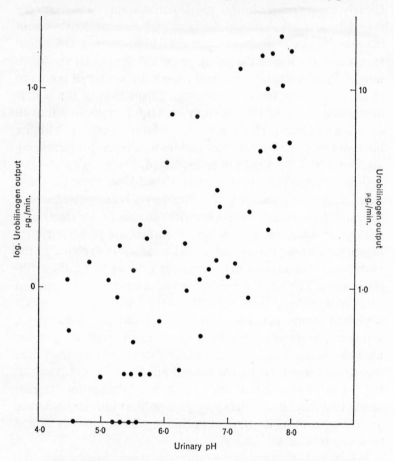

Reprinted from the *British Medical Journal*. Bourke E., Milne
M. D., and Stokes G. S. (1965), **2**, 1510. Mechanisms of renal
excretion of urobilinogen. (Table abbreviated.) (By permission
of the Authors, Editor, and Publishers.)

and log value 2·0 on the scale would be identical to the distance
between log value 0 and log value 1·0, i.e. equal vertical distances.
However, the natural number corresponding to log value 2·0 is

100, and this number would be marked on the extended right-hand scale opposite log value 2·0. On this scale, it is now observed that the vertical distance between 1·0 and 10 is the same as the vertical distance between 10 and 100. This is consistent with the statement that the vertical scale of the graph measures proportionate differences, since the ratios 100/10 and 10/1·0 are equal. Similarly if the reader picks out *any* three equally spaced points on a log scale, it will be found that the corresponding natural numbers represent equal proportionate differences.

The use of a logarithmic scale in Example 1.10 therefore implies that what is of interest is the relation between urinary pH value and proportionate changes in urobilinogen output. As a further illustration of this point consider the following hypothetical example:

Year	No. of subjects in screening programme
1970	5,000
1971	10,000
1972	20,000
1973	40,000

The absolute change in the number of subjects in the screening programme increases rapidly from year to year. The proportionate change from year to year is, however, constant at 100%. If two graphs of these data are drawn, one graph using an arithmetic scale and the other a logarithmic scale, and the two graphs superimposed, a marked difference in the appearance of the graphs will be seen (Fig. 1.3). Note that the log scale in Fig. 1.3 records the natural numbers corresponding to the log values on the scale, rather than the log values themselves. Comparison of the two scales in the figure also shows how the use of a log scale enables a much greater range of values to be recorded on a given size of graph.

In general logarithmic scales are used when there is interest in proportionate changes, or the *rate* of change in a variable, rather than in the absolute amount of change. There is nothing esoteric or complex about logarithmic or semi-logarithmic charts, but

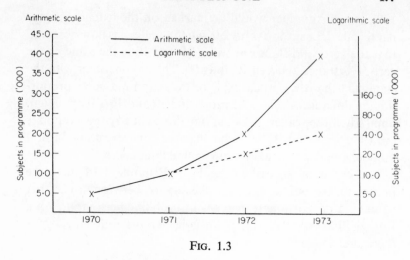

FIG. 1.3

they must be carefully interpreted. The important point to bear in mind is that a logarithmic scale measures proportionate or percentage changes in a variable.

1.4 Frequency distributions

In Fig. 1.4a below the histogram of Fig. 1.2 has been reproduced. An alternative method of presenting this frequency distribution is by means of a *frequency polygon* which in Fig. 1.4a has been superimposed on the histogram. In Fig. 1.4b the histogram has been removed. Examination of Fig. 1.4a will show how the frequency polygon is obtained. Straight lines join the mid-points of the top of each bar of the histogram.

The frequency polygon is constructed in such a way that the area enclosed by the polygon is equal to the area of the bars of the histogram. Earlier it was mentioned that the area of the bars of the histogram was proportional to the total frequency. It follows that the area enclosed by the frequency polygon is also proportional to the total frequency.

Having established this important point it is constructive to examine the shape of the frequency polygon itself. This consists of a series of straight lines and the terminal points of each line constitute the mid-points of the corresponding classes of the original frequency distribution. Thus, the peak of the polygon occurs above the value 27·5, which is the mid-point of the class with the greatest frequency. For various reasons which will later be made clear it would be convenient if the frequency polygon

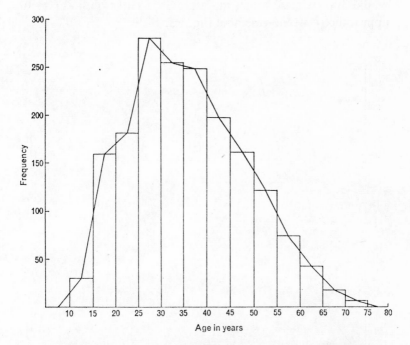

FIG. 1.4a. Histogram and superimposed frequency polygon of data in Example 1.2. Age distribution of 1,773 male Assam labour force

could be replaced by a smooth curve of approximately the same shape, and this can be done. To understand the reasoning behind this let us assume that the frequency distribution of Fig. 1.4a represents a sample from a very large or infinite population. Suppose now that a much larger sample is taken, say 20,000 rather than 1,773 and that the frequency distribution is organized in classes of 1 year instead of 5 years. The histogram of this distribution would in all likelihood be similar in shape to the earlier one and although there would be many more bars each bar would be much narrower in width, in fact one-fifth as wide. In the same way as before a frequency polygon could be drawn similar in shape to Fig. 1.4b. However, because the mid-points of each class were much closer together the frequency polygon would approximate much more closely to a smooth curve. In appearance it would resemble Fig. 1.5.

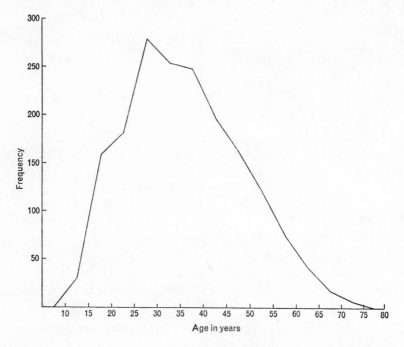

FIG. 1.4b. Frequency polygon

By taking larger and larger samples and by continually reducing the class interval the frequency polygon will approximate more and more closely to a smooth curve. The shape of the curve will depend upon the underlying frequency distribution for the whole population. Many distributions like the one discussed here rise to a peak and then decline.

Figure 1.6a is a symmetrical, bell-shaped, distribution. It can

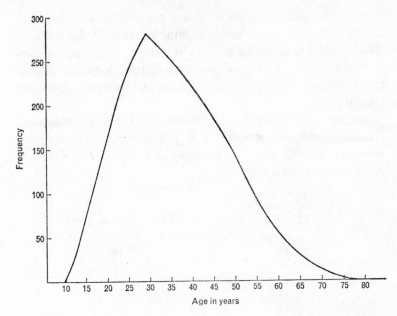

FIG. 1.5

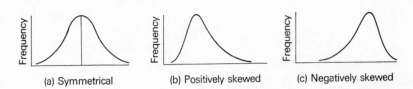

(a) Symmetrical   (b) Positively skewed   (c) Negatively skewed

FIG. 1.6. Types of frequency curve

be divided into two halves by the perpendicular drawn from the peak of the distribution and each half is a mirror image of the other half. Such a distribution which is very important in statistical analysis is called a *normal distribution*.

Figures 1.6b and 1.6c represent what are called *skewed* distributions. Such asymmetrical distributions are said to be positively or negatively skewed depending upon the direction of the 'tail' of the curve. Figure 1.6b is a *positively-skewed* distribution with a long tail at the upper end. Figure 1.6c is *negatively skewed*;

there is a long tail at the lower end of the distribution. Since the curves shown above are smooth continuous curves the variable, which is plotted along the horizontal scale, must also be assumed to be continuous. Curves of frequency distributions may assume any particular shape, of which the three illustrated above are special cases.

Another common form of frequency curve is the *cumulated frequency polygon*, or *ogive*. This will now be explained with reference to the data in Example 1.2. First, the data are rearranged in the following way:

Age (years) Less than	Cumulated frequency
15	30
20	190
25	372
30	651
35	905
40	1,153
45	1,350
50	1,511
55	1,632
60	1,706
65	1,749
70	1,767
75	1,773

The data have been rearranged by a process of successive cumulation of the frequencies in Example 1.2. Thus, 30 males are aged less than 15 years, 190 are aged less than 20 years $(30+160)$, 372 are aged less than 25 $(190+182)$, and so on. These are the cumulated frequencies. In Fig. 1.7, these cumulated frequencies have been plotted in the form of a cumulated frequency polygon, or ogive. When the points have been plotted, successive points are joined by straight lines. In principle, the ogive can be used to estimate the number of males aged less than a certain number of years, by interpolation. Suppose we wished to estimate the number of males aged less than 33; by erecting the ordinate from the relevant point on the horizontal scale, it can be estimated that about 800 males are aged less than 33 (see Fig. 1.7).

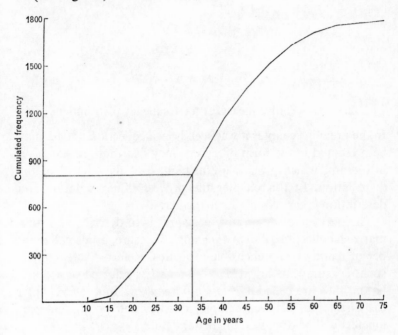

FIG. 1.7

2

2.1 Descriptive measures for frequency distributions

In the previous chapter it was seen how a collection of data may be presented in the form of a frequency distribution, such as a histogram, which gives a useful picture of the 'shape' of the distribution. In this chapter the process of presentation and description is carried one stage further.

The purpose of descriptive measures is to describe and summarize a collection of data by a single measure, or a small number of readily comprehensible measures. Referred to a sample, such measures are called *sample statistics*; referred to a population, they are called *population parameters*. In a later chapter the distinction between sample statistics and population parameters will be discussed in greater detail.

A variety of descriptive measures may be used to describe the same collection of data. Most readers are probably familiar with the idea of an 'average', which is used to describe the general level of magnitude of a particular variable. For example, it is common to refer to the average number of days spent in hospital by a given group of patients. There are a number of different ways in which the 'average' may be defined and measured and such a measure is called a *measure of central value* or *central location*.

A measure of central value, as its name suggests, 'locates' the middle or centre of a collection of values; sometimes, however, as will be seen, extreme values may also be of interest. A measure of central value may be used to divide observations into two equal groups, so that we may say, for example, half of a number of patients spend x days or less in hospital, and the remaining half spend x days or more in hospital. Other measures of location may be used to divide observations into two unequal groups;

thus, by calculating a measure of location called the *upper quartile*, it can be said that 75% of patients spend *y* days or less in hospital, and 25% spend *y* days or more. Similar measures of location may be used to 'locate' other points in a distribution of values, and in fact a measure of central value is merely a special type of measure of location.

Another type of measure frequently used in conjunction with a measure of central value is a *measure of dispersion*. The purpose of this measure will be explained more fully later in this chapter and in subsequent chapters; suffice it to say here that it is an extremely important measure which is used to describe the dispersion or variability of values in a distribution around their central value. Suppose, for example, it is calculated that the average weight of a number of patients is 180 lb, the way in which the individual weights are dispersed around this average may also be of interest. Do most of the patients' weights fall within the range 175–185 lb, or are they dispersed more widely around the average? A measure of dispersion provides a compact measure of the degree of dispersion of a group of values around the average.

Finally, *measures of skewness* will be briefly discussed. The notion of *positive* and *negative skewness* has already been mentioned in Chapter 1 and measures of skewness are designed to record the degree of skewness in a distribution.

2.2 Measures of central value

The most common measure of central value is the *arithmetic mean*; generally this is what is meant by the 'average' of a collection of values. The arithmetic mean of a number of observations is calculated by adding up the values of all the observations and dividing this total by the number of observations. The purpose of the arithmetic mean is to summarize a collection of data by means of a representative value—an average value.

The arithmetic mean is illustrated in Example 2.1 below, where the mean age of 20 patients on a chronic dialysis programme has been calculated. The symbol $\bar{X}$ stands for the arithmetic mean, and when used in future will refer to the arithmetic mean.

EXAMPLE 2.1

Clinical data of patients on chronic dialysis programme

Case no.	Age	Sex	Diagnosis
1	34	M	Chronic glomerulonephritis
2	33	M	Chronic glomerulonephritis. Malignant hypertension
3	24	M	Chronic glomerulonephritis. Malignant hypertension
4	34	F	Chronic pyelonephritis. Malignant hypertension
5	42	M	Polycystic kidneys
6	24	M	Chronic glomerulonephritis. Malignant hypertension
7	38	M	Chronic glomerulonephritis
8	31	M	Chronic pyelonephritis. Primary gout
9	36	M	Chronic glomerulonephritis. Malignant hypertension
10	25	M	Chronic glomerulonephritis. Malignant hyptertension
11	19	M	Chronic pyelonephritis
12	29	M	Chronic pyelonephritis
13	27	F	Chronic glomerulonephritis. Malignant hypertension
14	26	M	Chronic glomerulonephritis. Malignant hypertension
15	38	M	Chronic pyelonephritis
16	36	F	Chronic glomerulonephritis. Malignant hypertension
17	32	F	Chronic glomerulonephritis. Malignant hypertension
18	57	F	Polycystic kidneys
19	18	F	Chronic pyelonephritis
20	40	F	Chronic pyelonephritis

($\bar{X} = 643/20 = 32 \cdot 15$ years, i.e. the average age of the 20 patients.)

Reprinted from the *British Medical Journal.* Konotey-Ahulu F. I. D., Baillod R., Comty C. M., Heron J. R., Shaldon S., and Thomas P. K. (1965), **2**, 1212. Effect of periodic dialysis on the peripheral neuropathy of end-stage renal failure. (By permission of the Authors, Editor, and Publishers.)

In Example 2.1 it is particularly easy to calculate the arithmetic mean. The actual age of each patient is known and it is a simple matter to add up the individual ages and divide by 20. In Example 2.2 below, however, the data are presented in the form of a frequency distribution; the age of each patient is not known but only the age-group within which each patient falls. However, an estimate of the arithmetic mean age can still be made by making various assumptions. It is assumed that all 51 patients in the age-group 0–9 are aged 5 years exactly, that the 36 patients in the age-group 10–19 are aged 15 years exactly, and so on for each age-group. The values 5, 15, 25 and so on are the mid-points of the respective age-groups, as the reader may easily verify (remembering that the upper limit to the class 0–9, for example, is 9·999...); thus the mid-point of each class is taken as representative of the values within that class. In doing this it is not suggested that the 51 patients in the age-group 0–9 *are* aged 5 years exactly; it is suggested only that the *average* age of these 51 patients will be

EXAMPLE 2.2

Age distribution of the tracheostomies

Age group (years)	No. of tracheostomies
0–9	51
10–19	36
20–29	43
30–39	41
40–49	47
50–59	79
60–69	65
70–79	24
80+	3
Total	389

Reprinted from the *British Medical Journal.* McClelland R. M. A. (1965), **2**, 567. Complications of Tracheostomy (Table abbreviated.) (By permission of the Author, Editor, and Publishers.)

about 5 years and, since 5 is mid-way along the range of ages in this class, this seems a reasonable assumption to make.

One point to notice here is that the age-group 80-plus has no fixed upper limit, and therefore no fixed mid-point. All that can be done here is to arbitrarily assign an upper limit and then take a mid-point for the class. In the circumstances, we may reasonably take 90 as the upper class limit and 85 as the class mid-point— that is, the average age of the 3 patients in this age-group is assumed to be 85. Since the number of patients in this age-group is proportionately very small, any error in doing this would be very small also, although of course if all 3 patients happened to be 105 years old this could have a serious effect on our estimate of the overall arithmetic mean.

Using the method described above, the arithmetic mean age for this group of 389 patients is estimated as 41·3 years. Of course, since the actual age of each patient is not given this is only an estimate, but unless there is something peculiar about the distribution this estimated mean should be very close to the true (unknown) mean.*

The interpretation and use of the arithmetic mean requires little comment, since the concept of the 'average' is widely used and understood. The mean provides a useful summary measure for a particular collection of data, as in the examples above, and it is also useful for purposes of comparison. If, for instance, it is wished to compare the ages of the two groups of patients in Examples 2.1 and 2.2, the most convenient form of comparison is in terms of the average age of the two groups. Thus it can be said that, on average, a person in the first group is some 9–10 years younger than a person in the second group. Comparisons of this kind are very important in statistical analysis, and they will be discussed at greater length in a subsequent chapter.

Although the arithmetic mean is the most common measure of central value, there are several other measures which are widely

---

* Even in Example 2.1, however, there is an element of estimation involved, since age in each case is 'rounded off' and expressed as an integer. This element of estimation is involved in all cases where the variable concerned is continuous, like temperature, time, age.

used. One of these is the *median*. The median is the value of that observation which, when the observations are arranged in ascending order of magnitude, divides them into two equal groups. Consider the data shown in Example 2.3.

EXAMPLE 2.3

Consecutive readings on haemoscope, by different observers, of blood diluted 1:200 (as Oxyhaemoglobin)

Sample	1	2	3	4	5
Haemoscope readings	9·3	7·5	15·4	6·4	13·4
	9·2	6·9	15·8	6·0	14·2
	9·4	7·2	15·5	6·2	14·0
	10·0	7·6	15·5	6·2	13·8
	9·0	7·6	15·9	6·0	14·8
	9·9	7·7	16·0	6·4	13·2
	9·5	7·2	15·8	6·6	13·6
	9·2	8·2	15·8	6·0	13·8
	9·7	7·5	14·8	6·3	13·8
	9·4	7·5	15·3	6·0	13·5
	9·5	6·8	15·2	6·0	13·8
Mean	9·4	7·4	15·5	6·2	13·8
S.D.	0·31	0·39	0·36	0·21	0·43
Laboratory determination (by photoelectric color-imeter) as cyanmethae-moglobin	9·4	7·7	15·2	6·0	13·8

Reprinted from the *British Medical Journal*. Lewis S. M., and Carne S. J. (1965), **2**, 1167. Clinical haemoglobinometry: An evaluation of a modified Grey-Wedge photometer. (By permission of the Authors, Editor, and Publishers.)

For the moment we may ignore samples 2–5 and consider only the results of sample 1. Re-arranging the readings in this column in ascending order of magnitude, we have: 9·0, 9·2, 9·2, 9·3, 9·4, 9·4, 9·5, 9·5, 9·7, 9·9, 10·0. There are 11 observations altogether and so the middle observation is the 6th one. The value of the 6th observation, when the observations are arranged in order of magnitude, is 9·4 and so the median is 9·4. This can be obtained either by counting up from the bottom until the 6th lowest observation is reached, or counting down from the top until the 6th highest observation is reached.

The median age of patients can also be calculated for the data in Examples 2.1 and 2.2. In Example 2.1 there are 20 observations, which is an even number, and this is slightly more awkward because there is no single observation which can be unambiguously defined as the middle one. If the 10th observation is taken it is found that there are 10 observations above it (11–20) and 9 observations below it (1–9). The opposite holds true if the 11th observation is taken as the median. A solution is to take the median as mid-way between the values of the 10th and 11th observations, that is, as the average of the two middle observations. In Example 2.1, the 10th observation in ascending order of magnitude is 32, and the 11th observation is 33. The median is therefore 32·5 years. It can be said that the median exceeds in value not more than half the observations, and is exceeded in value by not more than half the observations.*

In Example 2.2 there are 389 observations and the median is the value of the 195th observation in ascending, or descending, order of magnitude. In this case the calculation is a little more complicated, since the exact age of each patient is not known but, as in the case of the arithmetic mean, the value of the median can be estimated with the aid of some simple assumptions. Referring back to the data in Example 2.2, it is clear that the 195th observation must lie in the age-group 40–49; there are 171 patients below the age of 40, and 218 patients below the age of 50, as the reader may verify by adding up the frequencies in the relevant age-groups. The problem now is to determine an exact value for the median within the 40–49 age-group, but this technical point will not be pursued here. In this particular example it happens

---

* If there are n observations, the median is the value of the $[(n + 1)/2]$th. observation. If n is odd, $(n + 1)/2$ will be an integer. If n is even, $(n + 1)/2$ will involve the fraction $\frac{1}{2}$.

that the estimated median value is exactly 45·0 years, which is |
also the mid-point of the class, but this is purely coincidental.

To summarize then, the median is calculated by arranging the
observations in ascending order of magnitude and the middle
value of the series is selected as representative of the average level
of magnitude of the variable. Thus, the median is an alternative
to the arithmetic mean as a measure of the average value for a
given group of observations.

Although the median is quite simple to calculate and commonly used as a measure of central value, the arithmetic mean is
generally preferred. The reasons for this will be dealt with later,
but at this stage it should be noted that in general, the arithmetic
mean and the median will be different in value. In Example 2.1 the
mean is 32·15 and the median is 32·5; in Example 2·2 the mean is
41·3 and the median is 45·0. Whether the median is less than,
greater than, or in rare cases equal to the mean depends upon the
general shape and characteristics of the particular distribution
concerned, a point which will be discussed later in this chapter.
However for many types of distribution the mean and the median
will be fairly close in value, and the median is also a useful
measure of central value.

A third measure of central value is the *mode*. The mode may
be defined as the most commonly occurring value, or as the value
of the variable which occurs with the greatest frequency. An
example of the mode arises from the experiment of Carne and
Lewis, quoted in Example 2.3. Re-arranging the readings in
sample 4 (Example 2.3) in ascending order of magnitude, we have
6·0, 6·0, 6·0, 6·0, 6·0, 6·2, 6·2, 6·3, 6·4, 6·4, 6·6. The arithmetic
mean for this sample, to one place of decimals is 6·2, and the
median value is also 6·2. It might be argued, however, that a more
representative value for these readings is 6·0, since this value
occurs in almost half the observations; as the most commonly
occurring value, 6·0 is also the modal value of this distribution.
From this point of view, the mode might be considered a more
useful representative or average value for the distribution, even
though in this particular case the mode is not located in the middle
of the series of observations.

The mode of a frequency distribution, such as that in Example 2.2, can also be calculated. It may be remembered that in the previous chapter it was explained how a frequency distribution may be illustrated by means of a histogram and a frequency polygon. It was observed also that as the number of observations is increased, and the class intervals are reduced, the frequency polygon approaches more and more closely a smooth unbroken curve. The point at which this curve reaches a peak represents the maximum frequency, and the value which corresponds to this maximum frequency is the mode.

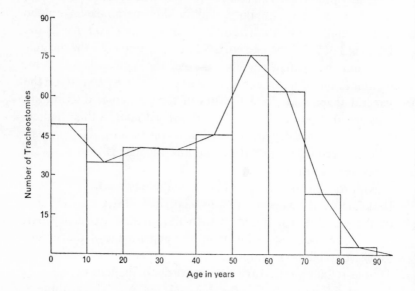

FIG. 2.1. Histogram and frequency polygon of the data in Example 2.2

Figure 2.1 shows the histogram and frequency polygon which corresponds to the distribution of Example 2.2. For simplicity the age-group 80-plus is taken to be 80 and under 90. It will be observed that the peak of the distribution, or the point of maximum frequency, occurs in the age-group 50 and under 60. More patients fall into this age-group than into any other. It can be said, therefore, that 50 and under 60 is the *modal age-group* or, more generally, the *modal class*. Suppose more and more observations are taken and the class interval is reduced, then as the frequency polygon approached a smooth curve, the peak of the curve would be expected to occur somewhere in the range 50 and under 60. On the basis of the information provided, it cannot be determined precisely where this hypothetical peak will occur but, as for the mean and the median, its position can be estimated. This position will provide us with an estimate of the modal value.

In general, the procedure is first to determine the modal class and then to determine algebraically an exact value for the mode within that class. This latter step need not detain us here. In the example the value of the mode is estimated as 56·9 years. That is, 56·9 years is assumed to be the value at which the hypothetical curve corresponding to the distribution of Example 2.2 is at a maximum. In the sense that the mode is the most frequently occurring value, it may be said to be a representative or average value, and may also be used as a measure of central value like the mean or the median. For reasons explained in a later section of this chapter, the mode is usually different in value from both the mean and the median.

As a measure of central value the mode is less commonly used than either the arithmetic mean or the median. Moreover some distributions do not have a modal value, while other distributions may have more than one modal value.

There is one further measure of central value which will be discussed here. This is the *geometric mean* and it is illustrated in Example 2.4. The values of the arithmetic mean and median are also given, for comparative purposes. As explained, the arithmetic mean is calculated by adding up all the values in the distribution and dividing the resulting total by the number of observations, in this case 66. The geometric mean is calculated by adding up all the logarithm values of the variable, dividing the total by the number of observations (66), and taking the anti-log of the answer.

This may be thought a rather peculiar method of calculating an

EXAMPLE 2.4

Residues in human fat (parts per million)

Sex	Total B.H.C.	Dieldrin	Origin
F	0·1	0·2	—
M	Trace	0·1	—
F	0·2	0·2	Cardiff
M	0·5	0·15	Liverpool
M	0·3	Trace	—
M	0·3	0·15	—
M	0·2	0·1	Newcastle
M	0·2	0·1	Carlisle
F	0·4	0·1	London
M	0·2	0·1	London
F	0·3	0·1	Carlisle
M	0·1	0·2	Carlisle
M	0·3	Trace	London
M	0·3	0·1	Carlisle
M	0·4	0·1	—
F	0·6	0·2	Newcastle
F	0·6	0·2	London
F	0·5	0·15	Carlisle
F	0·2	0·1	London
F	Trace	Trace	Carlisle
M	0·7	0·1	London
M	0·5	0·2	Carlisle
F	0·4	0·2	Newcastle
F	0·7	0·4	London
M	0·2	0·25	—
F	0·3	0·2	Bolton
M	0·3	Trace	Carlisle
M	0·2	0·2	London
M	0·6	0·4	London
M	0·9	0·3	Cardiff
F	0·5	0·3	Cardiff
F	0·1	0·3	Leeds
M	0·7	0·8	London
M	0·4	0·1	Newcastle
M	Trace	0·2	London
F	0·3	0·1	London
M	1·0	0·9	London
M	0·3	0·2	Cardiff

EXAMPLE 2.4—*continued*

M	0·5	0·4	London
M	0·5	0·4	London
M	0·4	0·3	Leeds
M	0·5	0·3	Leeds
M	0·8	0·7	London
M	0·4	0·3	Cardiff
M	0·1	0·1	Bolton
F	0·5	0·2	London
F	1·0	0·4	London
M	0·7	0·4	London
M	0·4	0·5	Cardiff
M	0·8	0·4	Portsmouth
F	0·5	0·3	—
M	0·6	0·4	Carlisle
M	0·2	0·1	Cardiff
M	0·3	0·3	Bolton
M	0·4	0·1	Cardiff
F	0·5	0·5	London
F	0·3	0·25	—
M	0·3	0·2	Newcastle
F	0·3	0·2	Portsmouth
M	0·7	0·2	London
M	0·9	0·8	Cardiff
F	0·6	0·3	Carlisle
M	0·3	0·3	Carlisle
F	0·3	0·3	Bournemouth
M	0·3	0·1	Bolton
M	0·5	0·3	Cardiff

Mean pesticide-residue levels in human fat (all
levels are expressed in parts per million)

	Total B.H.C.	Dieldrin
Mean value	0·42	0·26
Median value	0·39	0·18
Geometric mean	0·34	0·21

Reprinted from the *British Medical Journal*. Egan H., Goulding
R., Roburn J., and Tatton J. O'G. (1965), **2**, 66. Organo-chlorine
pesticide residues in human fat and human milk. (Tables abbreviated.) (By permission of the Authors, Editor, and Publishers.)

average. However, sometimes the geometric mean is a more
appropriate measure to use than the arithmetic mean, for instance
in averaging ratios or for distributions which are markedly
skewed. Since the geometric mean is the average of the logarithm
values of a series of observations, it is appropriate to use in cases
where data are transformed logarithmically, as in Example 1.10.
√ The geometric mean is always less than the arithmetic mean in
value.

Four different measures of central value have now been
described. At this stage it may occur to the reader that the concept
of an 'average' or 'central value' is not at all precise, and this is in
fact the case. Each of the measures described may be claimed to
be an 'average' in some sense, and yet they will generally be
different in value when used to describe the same data. Yet this
is less confusing than it may seem, because the same ambiguities
occur when the word 'average' is used in normal conversation,
even though one may be quite clear what is meant when the term
is used. If for instance it is said that the 'average' number of
children per family in Ireland is 2, this does not mean that it is the
precise arithmetic mean, which may be 2·7 or 3·6. What is meant
is that 2 is the most commonly occurring family size—that more
families have two children than those with one or three, for
example. In this case the mode is being used as the 'average'
value. In contrast, if it is said that the average age of the Irish
male population is 32·4 years, probably the arithmetic mean age
is being referred to. Or again, if it was decided to say something
about the average income of medical practitioners, the median
might be preferred, for this will indicate that half the doctors in a
survey earn the median income or less and half earn the median
income or more. In general, no hard and fast rules can be laid
down about which measure to use—any one of the measures may
be the most suitable in a particular instance. The mean, median
and mode may be close together in value, or they may differ
considerably in value; this depends upon the shape of the
distribution, to which reference will be made later. As already
mentioned, the arithmetic mean is the most commonly used
measure, and unless there are specific reasons for not using the

arithmetic mean this measure is to be preferred in data which is ⌞
symmetrically distributed; it follows that in asymmetrical distributions the geometric mean, median, and mode are generally
more appropriate measures of central value. However, the
purpose of all four measures is the same—it is to describe or
summarize a collection of data by means of an average or
representative value.

2.3   Other measures of location

All the measures so far discussed are measures of central value;
that is, they are designed to 'locate' the centre or middle of a
distribution. However, it may also be of interest to locate other
points in the distribution. Consider the data in Example 2.5
which is based on the frequency distribution of Example 2.2
on p. 25.

EXAMPLE 2.5

Median, quartiles and percentiles of the age distribution of tracheostomies

	Age in years
10th percentile	7·6
Lower quartile (25th percentile)	22·4
Median (50th percentile)	45·0
Upper quartile (75th percentile)	59·3
90th percentile	68·2

These data may be interpreted as follows; the median, which
has already been explained, divides the distribution into two
halves. Thus 50% of patients are aged 45·0 or over, and 50% are
aged 45·0 or less. For this reason the median may be described as
the *50th percentile*. Other percentiles may be similarly interpreted.
Thus the 10th percentile (7·6) divides the distribution into two
groups; 10% of the patients are aged 7·6 years or less, and 90%
are aged 7·6 or more. Similarly the 25th percentile shows us that
25% of the patients are 22·4 years or less, and that 75% are aged

22·4 or more. Like the 50th percentile, the 25th percentile has a special name; it is called the *lower quartile*.

The *upper quartile* and *90th percentile* are clearly the 'mirror images' in the upper half of the distribution of the lower quartile and 10th percentile respectively and may be correspondingly interpreted by the reader. The 90th percentile is sometimes called the 'upper 10th percentile'. The measures included in the example and their interpretation should illustrate, without requiring formal definitions, the meaning and purpose of percentiles. Percentiles are used to divide a distribution into convenient groups; the median, which is the most important percentile value, divides the distribution in half. The next two most important percentile values are the lower and upper quartiles, which divide the distribution into groups in the ratio $1:3$ and $3:1$ respectively. Other percentile values can be calculated, for example the 20th percentile, or the 69th percentile, but those shown in the example are the most important. Quartiles and other percentile values are calculated in a manner similar to that used for the calculation of the median.

The median 'locates', either exactly or by estimation, the middle value in a distribution. The quartiles and other percentiles similarly locate other points or values in the distribution. All these measures are called measures of location. The median, like the mean and the mode, is a special (i.e. particularly important), measure of location, and is called a measure of central value or central location. Whilst measures of central location are the most important, other measures of location assist in describing a distribution more fully. In certain circumstances measures like the lower quartile or the 90th percentile may be of greater interest than the median. For example, in the occurrence of tracheostomies amongst younger people (Example 2.2) it may be useful to know that 25% of the tracheostomies were performed on persons under the age of 23. By using the median in conjunction with other measures such as the quartiles, a compact description of the distribution can be obtained.

2.4 Measures of dispersion

In Example 2.3, data concerning consecutive readings by different observers on a haemoscope were shown. These data are reproduced in Example 2.6.

EXAMPLE 2.6

Consecutive readings on haemoscope, by different observers, of blood diluted 1:200 (as oxyhaemoglobin)

Sample	1	2	3	4	5
Haemoscope readings	9·3	7·5	15·4	6·4	13·4
	9·2	6·9	15·8	6·0	14·2
	9·4	7·2	15·5	6·2	14·0
	10·0	7·6	15·5	6·2	13·8
	9·0	7·6	15·9	6·0	14·8
	9·9	7·7	16·0	6·4	13·2
	9·5	7·2	15·8	6·6	13·6
	9·2	8·2	15·8	6·0	13·8
	9·7	7·5	14·8	6·3	13·8
	9·4	7·5	15·3	6·0	13·5
	9·5	6·8	15·2	6·0	13·8
Mean	9·4	7·4	15·5	6·2	13·8
S.D.	0·31	0·39	0·36	0·21	0·43
Laboratory determination (by photoelectric colorimeter) as cyanmethaemoglobin	9·4	7·7	15·2	6·0	13·8

Reprinted from the *British Medical Journal*. Lewis S. M., and Carne S. J. (1965), **2**, 1167. Clinical haemoglobinometry: An evaluation of a modified Grey-Wedge photometer. (By permission of the Authors, Editor, and Publishers.)

The third last line of the table is the arithmetic mean reading for each sample. The main interest in this experiment, however, lies in the *variation* in individual readings, and the values of the standard deviation shown in the second last line of the table are designed to measure the degree of variation or dispersion in each sample.

The standard deviation is the most important measure of dispersion used in statistical analysis, and is worth considering in some detail. Consider, for example, sample 4, for which the arithmetic mean is 6·2. It is observed, as expected, that the individual readings in the sample are dispersed around the arithmetic mean. In this particular sample, with the exception of one reading of 6·6, they are closely concentrated around the arithmetic mean. It would be convenient to describe this dispersion of values around the arithmetic mean by means of a single compact measure, and this is in fact the purpose of the standard deviation. The difference between any individual reading and the arithmetic mean is called a deviation, and the standard deviation is a kind of average of the individual deviations. Thus in sample 4 the deviation between the first reading (6·4) and the mean is 0·2, the deviation between the second reading (6·0) and the mean is −0·2, and so on. The standard deviation of the eleven values in sample 4 is given as 0·21, and this may be described as a measure of the average dispersion of the eleven values around their arithmetic mean. Comparing the value of the standard deviation with the variation of individual values around the arithmetic mean, it is not difficult to grasp the concept of the standard deviation as a measure of average dispersion or deviation.

At this point an important property of the arithmetic mean may be mentioned. This is, that the sum of deviations from the arithmetic mean is zero. For example, the arithmetic mean of the four numbers 4, 6, 8, and 10 is 7, and the deviations of values from the arithmetic mean are −3, −1, 1, and 3 respectively. The minus deviations cancel out the plus deviations; as a result, the standard deviation cannot be calculated algebraically as the average of the deviations, whose sum is always zero. (If the reader checks sample 4 it will be found that the sum of the deviations from the mean is not exactly zero; this is because the mean has been expressed to one place of decimals only.) In calculating the dispersion of values around the arithmetic mean, however, it is immaterial whether the deviations are plus or minus; only the numerical magnitude of the deviation is of interest. Hence, to avoid getting zero when the deviations are added together, the individual deviations are squared, to eliminate the minus signs. The average of these squared deviations is called the *variance*, and the square root of the variance is the *standard deviation*. As a result of this method of calculation, the standard deviation is sometimes referred to as the *root mean square deviation*.

Returning to sample 4, the square of the first deviation (0·2) is 0·04, and the square of the second (−0·2) is also 0·04. Continuing this process, the square of each deviation is obtained, and the squared deviations added up. In sample 4 the sum of squares of the deviations is 0·45, the average* of this sum of squares is 0·045 (the variance), and the standard deviation is readily calculated as $\sqrt{0\cdot045} = 0\cdot21$.

For comparative purposes it is useful now to consider sample 5. Here the mean is 13·8 and, by inspection, it is clear that there is a greater dispersion of values around the mean, than in the case of sample 4. Thus the deviation of the first reading (13·4) from the mean is −0·4, the deviation of the second reading is 0·4, and the deviation of the fifth reading (14·8) from the mean is as great as 1·0. For this reason it is to be expected that the standard deviation will be higher for sample 5 than for sample 4, and this is so: it is 0·43.

The standard deviation, then, can be interpreted as a measure of the dispersion of values around their central value. In the particular example above, the value of the standard deviation is more important than the value of the arithmetic mean. The object of the experiment is to determine the degree of variation in readings by different observers, and the standard deviation provides a measure of this variation. The arithmetic mean and the standard deviation are complementary measures. The arithmetic mean measures the general level of magnitude of the distribution, or its central value; the standard deviation shows how

---

* For reasons which need not be discussed here, the sum of the squared deviations is divided by N − 1 rather than N (where N is the number of observations) to obtain the variance. Thus in the example given the sum of the squares of the deviations is divided by ten, rather than eleven, to obtain the variance.

closely the individual values in the distribution are dispersed around the central value. The greater the range of values in a particular distribution, the greater the value of the standard deviation. In illustration of this point, the reader should examine the means and standard deviations of the five samples in Example 2.6.

Frequent references to the standard deviation and its properties are made in subsequent chapters of this book, and the reader should make a special effort to grasp the meaning of this measure. The variance and standard deviation may also be calculated for a frequency distribution, such as that of Example 2.2. As for the mean, the calculation is somewhat longer for a grouped distribution, but the method of calculation is the same as for ungrouped data.

Other measures of dispersion are available. The *mean deviation* is calculated by ignoring the minus signs in the individual deviations, adding the deviations together, and taking the average. Thus, the mean deviation for sample 4 in Example 2.3 is 0·17. The *quartile deviation* (or semi-interquartile range) is calculated as half the difference between the upper and lower quartiles. Thus the quartile deviation for the distribution of Example 2.2 may be calculated (see Example 2.5) as $(59·3 - 22·4)/2 = 18·45$ years. However, these alternative measures of dispersion are not frequently used.

In summary, measures of dispersion are designed to show how closely the values in a distribution are grouped around their central value. If there is a considerable variation or range of values in a distribution, one should expect a relatively high value for the measure of dispersion. At the other extreme, if all the values in a distribution were equal, then the measure of dispersion would be zero.

2.5 Measures of skewness

It may be recalled that skewness was mentioned in the previous chapter, in connection with curves of frequency distributions. In Fig. 2.2 three types of frequency distribution are illustrated.

As already explained in Chapter 1, Fig. 2.2a represents a symmetrical distribution, Fig. 2.2b represents a positively skewed distribution, and Fig. 2.2c represents a negatively skewed distribution.

For most purposes it is sufficient to know the direction of skewness; that is, whether the distribution is positively or negatively skewed, or symmetrical. Sometimes however it is desirable to be more precise, and to attempt to measure the degree or amount of skewness.

There are several ways in which skewness can be measured. The simplest method, called the Pearsonian measure of skewness, will be considered here. This measure is based upon the difference between the arithmetic mean and the mode. In Fig. 2.2a it will be noticed that the mean and the mode are equal in value, and this

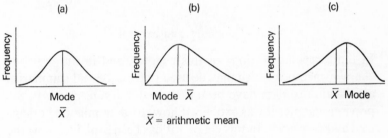

FIG. 2.2

is characteristic of a symmetrical distribution. In a positively skewed distribution, the mean always lies to the right of the mode, as Fig. 2.2b shows. In a negatively skewed distribution, the mean is always below the mode, as illustrated by Fig. 2.2c. The Pearsonian measure of skewness is calculated as

$$\frac{Mean - Mode}{Standard\ Deviation}$$

In Fig. 2.2a the difference between the mean and the mode is zero and hence the measure of skewness is zero. In Fig. 2.2b the difference (Mean–Mode) is some positive amount and the measure of skewness will be a positive value. In Fig. 2.2c the difference (Mean–Mode) will be negative and the measure of skewness will therefore be a negative value. (The standard deviation is always positive.)

The value of the measure of skewness therefore depends upon the difference between the mean and the mode. In a normal distribution the mean and the mode coincide. The greater the degree of skewness in a distribution, the greater will be the difference between the mean and the mode and hence the greater the value of the measure of skewness. This value gives some idea of how skewed the distribution is, whilst the algebraic sign of the measure indicates whether the skewness is positive or negative. Values numerically greater than $+1$ or -1 are unusual.

It is generally important to know whether or not a distribution is skewed and if so whether it is in a positive or negative direction, but for ordinary purposes a numerical measure of skewness is seldom required.

2.6 Summary and examples

In the foregoing sections of this chapter, and in the previous chapter, methods which may be used to describe and summarize a collection of data have been discussed and illustrated. In the previous chapter it was explained how the data might be organized and presented. In this chapter it has been explained how the important characteristics of a distribution may be summarized by means of measures of location, measures of dispersion, and measures of skewness.

In Example 2.7 below, various measures, discussed in this chapter, have been used to describe and compare two distributions and by now the reader will be familiar with the meaning and interpretation of the descriptive measures used. The statistics are useful to describe the salient features of each distribution and they enable the reader to see at a glance the principal points of difference or similarity.

Both distributions are positively skewed, the anti-tetanus serum more so than the tetanus toxoid. The former distribution also shows a greater dispersion of values around the arithmetic mean, as measured by the standard deviation. Since the distributions are positively skewed, in both cases the mean is greater than the mode. It will also be noticed that in both examples the

EXAMPLE 2.7

Number of patients given anti-tetanus serum and
tetanus toxoid, by age and sex

Age (years)	Anti-tetanus serum Both sexes	Tetanus toxoid Both sexes
0–9	844	8
10–19	856	8
20–29	280	271
30–39	217	257
40–49	212	145
50–59	198	37
60–69	97	3
70–79	20	—
80–89	2	—
All ages	2,726	729

Reprinted from the *British Journal of Preventive and Social Medicine*. Binns P. M. (1961), **15**, 180. An analysis of tetanus prophylaxis in 3,455 cases. (Table abbreviated.) (By permission of the Author, Editor, and Publishers.)

Measure	Anti-tetanus serum	Tetanus toxoid
Arithmetic mean	22·0	33·9
Median	16·1	33·0
Mode	10·2	29·5
Upper quartile	33·0	40·2
Lower quartile	8·1	26·1
Standard deviation	18·2	9·6
Pearsonian measure of skewness	0·65	0·45

median is greater than the mode but less than the mean, and this is also characteristic of positively skewed distributions. In negatively skewed distributions the order of these three measures is reversed; the mean is less than the median, which in turn is less than the mode, while in a symmetrical distribution, the mean, median and mode are all equal.

D

3

3.1 Samples and populations

At the beginning of the previous chapter mention was made of a *sample* and a *population* and a distinction was noted between *sample statistics* and *population parameters*. Now the distinction between samples and populations will be examined in greater detail. The basic statistical concepts discussed here are essential to an understanding of the following chapters and the reader is advised to study this chapter carefully. It will be noted that summaries are interspersed throughout the chapter. These summaries will assist the reader and will eliminate the need for referring to preceding pages.

The term 'population' is used here in a technical sense to describe all the observations or units of a particular variable or attribute. One can refer to a population of doctors, a population of ages of Irishmen at death, or a population of readings on a haemoscope. What is to be understood as the 'population' varies according to the context in which it is used. Thus, the population of doctors in Dublin and the population of doctors in the whole of Ireland are quite distinct populations. It is then important to understand that the term 'the population' has a precise meaning in any given context.

A population may be *finite* or *infinite*. The population of hospital patients in Ireland at or over any particular period of time is finite. On the other hand, the population of readings on a haemoscope or a thermometer is infinite since, in principle, an indefinite number of such readings can be taken. Many populations are so large that they may be regarded as infinite—for example, the number (population) of red blood cells in the human body.

44

In its broadest sense a sample refers to any specific collection of observations drawn from a parent population. We may have a sample of doctors, a sample of temperature readings, and so on. At one extreme the sample may include all the units in the parent population, in which case it is referred to as a *full count* or *census*.* A full count is only possible, of course, if the population is finite. At the other extreme a sample may consist of only one unit selected from the population.

In a narrower sense a sample implies a collection of observations which have been selected in a particular way from the population. Various methods may be used to select such a sample from a population. The reader is probably familiar with the notion of a *simple random sample* which is the best-known type of sample. Briefly, this is a sample selected in such a way that each unit or observation in the population has an equal chance of selection. This is the principle used in the selection of winning tickets in a lottery, or in the selection of prize-winning Premium Bonds or Prize Bonds. This and other types of sample design will be mentioned later in this chapter. It is sufficient to state at this point that, in general, the object in selecting a sample is to obtain a *representative* selection of units or observations from the parent population.

The relationship between samples and populations is fundamental to statistical analysis. When data are collected on a particular topic a first step is to describe and summarize the data by means of the techniques outlined in the previous two chapters. Generally, however, such data will represent a sample of observations from a certain population and the ultimate aim of the analysis of the data will be to infer something about the whole population on the basis of the sample. Suppose, for example, a random sample of persons 65 years of age and over living in a certain area reveals that the average weekly income of those included in the sample is £10.50, and that 20% of those in the

* The term 'census' refers to a full count of the specific population, i.e. all the units in the population are included. An example is a national population census. The term 'sample census' is sometimes used to refer to a sample selected from a specific population.

sample receive less than £6.00 per week. On the basis of the information collected in this sample it may be reasonable to infer
that the average weekly income of *all* persons 65 years of age and
over living in the area is £10.50, and that 20 % of *all* such persons
receive less than £6.00 per week. The validity of this inference
depends, of course, on the extent to which the sample is representative of the whole population of persons 65 years of age and
over living in the particular area. This will be further discussed
in a following section. In summary such a sample is of interest
because it may be used to provide information about the whole
of a particular population without the necessity of examining
every unit in that population.

It is now necessary to explain the difference and relationship
between sample statistics and population parameters. In the
previous chapter it was explained how various measures such as
the mean and the standard deviation could be used to describe
and summarize data. When these measures are applied to a
sample they are referred to as sample statistics or in the singular
as a sample statistic; the mean is usually written as $\bar{X}$ or $\bar{x}$ and the
standard deviation as s. When these measures are used to describe
a population they are referred to as population parameters and
then the mean is written as μ (mu) and the standard deviation as σ
(sigma).* Let us assume that the mean birth-weight of all liveborn
babies in Ireland in 1973 is 6·8 lb and that the standard deviation
is 1·9 lb. Since these measures refer to the population of birth-
weights in 1973 they may be written as $\mu = 6\cdot8$ lb, $\sigma = 1\cdot9$ lb.
Now suppose a random sample of 50 of these births is selected
and the mean and standard deviation weight calculated for this
sample. It is most unlikely that the mean weight for the sample
would be exactly 6·8 lb, or that the standard deviation would be
exactly 1·9 lb, for it cannot be expected that the sample will
exactly reflect the population from which it was drawn. On the

* However, while the standard deviation of a population is almost invariably
written as σ, it is not uncommon to find the standard deviation of a *sample*
written as σ, which is rather confusing, or as $\tilde{\sigma}$. It is usually clear from the
context whether the standard deviation of the sample or the population is
being referred to.

other hand, given the known variation in birth-weights it would be surprising if the mean of the sample were as high as 9·0 lb, or as low as 5·0 lb. If asked to hazard a guess one might claim to be 'reasonably confident' that the mean birth-weight of 50 babies randomly selected from the population would lie somewhere between 6·0 and 7·5 lb. A statement of this kind does, in fact, involve an application of the principles of statistical inference; and in the following sections it will be explained how much more precise statements of this kind can be made concerning the relationship between sample statistics and population parameters.

Returning to the hypothetical example quoted above, suppose the mean birth-weight for the sample of 50 births was 7·0 lb, and the standard deviation 1·8 lb. This can be written, $\bar{X} = 7·0$ lb, $s = 1·8$ lb. The sample statistics are not exactly equal to the population parameters but they are close to them in value; in a general sense the sample statistics may be said to be 'consistent' with the population parameters. Similarly, if another random sample of 50 birth-weights was taken one would expect the mean of this sample also to be close to 6·8 lb. Repeating the procedure a whole series of samples of size 50 could be collected and sample means calculated. Some of these sample means would be equal to the population mean in value but most of them would differ slightly from the population mean.*

Let us now summarize what has been said. The mean and standard deviation of a random sample of size N will generally be different from the mean and standard deviation of the population from which the sample was drawn. However, to the extent that a random sample reflects its parent population the sample mean will be close to the population mean in value and repeated samples of size N will generate a series of sample means which will be clustered within a certain range around the population mean.

In the following two sections these general statements concerning the relationship between sample statistics and population

---

* Sampling may be with or without replacement. It is assumed, throughout this chapter, that sampling is with replacement; that is, the units selected in one sample are replaced before the next sample is taken.

parameters are elaborated and the objectives of sampling are explained.

3.2   The normal distribution

The objectives of sampling are—(a) to make inferences about the population from which the sample is drawn, and (b) to test hypotheses about the population from which the sample is drawn. These two very similar applications of statistical inference may be respectively referred to as *estimation*, and *testing hypotheses*.

Under the first heading (estimation) the aim is to make statements about the population on the basis of the results of a sample. More precisely, it is required to estimate the value of certain population parameters such as the mean and standard deviation. In many instances the values of the population parameters are unknown and sample statistics are used to estimate the values of the corresponding population parameters. Suppose, for example, it was required to estimate the average height of all Irishmen 21 years of age and over. It would be impractical to measure every unit (man) in the population and instead a sample would be used. If a sufficiently large random sample is taken, the sample mean will be a 'good estimate' of the population mean. The given sample mean may not be exactly equal to the (unknown) population mean, but it will be possible to claim with reasonable confidence that the population mean will lie within a certain range on either side of the sample mean. The notion of using a sample in this way to infer something about a population is probably familiar to most readers, even to those without any knowledge of statistical method. As explained in the previous section the means of repeated random samples of the same size drawn from a given population will be distributed closely around the population mean. For reasons that will be explained shortly we can go further than this and state that almost all sample means will lie within a certain range of the population mean. Conversely, it follows from this that in almost all cases the population mean will lie within a certain range of any one sample mean. Thus, suppose that the mean height of a random sample of 100 Irishmen 21 years of age and over is found to be 68 in. Then, on the basis of this information a statement such as 'the mean height of all Irishmen 21 years of age and over lies within the range 68 ± 0·5 in.' may be made. Exactly how this estimate for the population mean is determined will be explained in a moment.

Under the second heading (testing hypotheses), the aim is to determine whether the results of a sample are consistent with certain assumed characteristics of the population, or whether the results of different samples are consistent with one another. For example, suppose it was asserted that the mean height of Irishmen 21 years of age and over was 69 in. and the mean of a sample of 50 of these men was found to be 67·5. Does the sample result support the hypothesis that the population mean is 69 in?

As already stated the means of repeated random samples of size N drawn from a population will be distributed within a certain range on either side of the population mean. For example, if repeated samples of size N are drawn from the population, it can be established, subject to certain conditions explained below, that 95% of the means of these samples will lie within a certain range of the population mean (μ). Similarly, a range can be calculated which will include 99% of all sample means. Hence if a given sample mean ($\bar{X}$) lies within the 95% range it may be said to be 'consistent' with the population mean.

Suppose a particular sample mean ($\bar{X}$) is calculated and found to lie outside the range within which we expect 95% of the sample means to lie. One explanation for this may be that since the specified range claims to account for only 95% of the sample means, we may have selected, by chance, one of the 5% of sample means which lie outside this range. This is quite possible. Another explanation is that the sample is not a random sample— it is biased in some way; for example, tall men may have been deliberately or accidentally excluded from the sample. A third explanation is that the statement or hypothesis is incorrect—the sample has not been drawn from a population with mean μ.

If the first and second events can be excluded then the conclusion which emerges is that the sample mean is 'inconsistent' with the population mean. With reference to the example quoted this would be interpreted as indicating that a sample mean of 67·5 in. is inconsistent with an assumed population mean of 69 in.; if the population mean *is* 69 in., we should not expect to get a sample mean as different from this as 67·5 in. A more detailed example of this type of test will be given shortly.

The tests outlined above are not confined to estimates, or tests of hypotheses, of means. Other population parameters such as the standard deviation, for example, may also be estimated or tested on the basis of sample results. The range of application of tests based on the principles of statistical inference is very wide and many complex methods of analysis have been developed to deal with a variety of statistical problems; some of these are referred to in later chapters. All these techniques depend upon certain basic principles of statistical inference and the remainder of this section is devoted to a more detailed, but nevertheless elementary, explanation of these principles. A firm understanding of the types of test described below will enable the reader to understand the logic and purpose of other tests referred to in the following chapters. The tests described now will be confined to the relationship between population means and sample means and will cover estimation, and testing hypotheses.

A general outline of the relationship between a population mean and the means of random samples of a certain size drawn from that population has been given above. Suppose again that we have a very large or infinite population with a mean value of μ, and a standard deviation of σ. Now suppose a random sample of size N (N fairly large, say 50) is drawn from this population, and the sample mean ($\bar{X}$) calculated. In general $\bar{X}$ and μ will be different for reasons already explained. Suppose further samples of size N are drawn from this population and a series of sample means are calculated. If a hundred such samples were collected there would be a hundred sample means; some of these would be greater than the population mean μ, and others would be less.

An important result may now be stated. *The mean of all these sample means will come closer to μ, as the number of samples increases.* Since each sample mean is an approximation of the population mean and since the sample means are distributed around the population mean this seems a reasonable proposition. To give this statement more concrete form, suppose 10 random samples of 50 males 21 years of age and over are taken; the 10 sample means will vary amongst themselves, and from the population mean (μ), but *the mean of the 10 sample means* will lie very close to μ, and will be a good estimate of the mean height of all adult males, i.e. the population mean.

If 100 samples are selected from a population the sample means may be presented in the form of a frequency distribution. In turn, this frequency distribution may be illustrated in the form of a histogram and frequency polygon. Now, it has already been explained in a previous chapter that as the number of observations is increased and the class intervals are reduced a frequency polygon approaches a smooth curve. Similarly, if repeated samples of size N are drawn from a population and the distribution of these sample means is shown by constructing a frequency polygon, then as the number of sample means increases and the class intervals are reduced this frequency polygon will eventually approach a smooth curve. This curve is called the probability distribution of sample means or the *sampling distribution of the mean*.

In the three preceding paragraphs it has been explained: (1) that the means of repeated random samples drawn from a population will be distributed around the population mean; (2) as the number of samples increases the mean of the sample means will come closer to μ, the population mean; (3) that the distribution of sample means around the population mean may be illustrated by a smooth curve, called the sampling distribution of the mean. The exact shape of any sampling distribution of the mean depends upon a number of factors, including the size and degree of skewness of the population from which the samples are drawn, and the size of those samples. However, for large samples (say greater than 50) it can be shown that in many cases the sampling distribution of the mean is a symmetrical, bell-shaped distribution, whose central value is the population mean μ. Such a distribution has already been referred to in previous chapters as a *normal curve* or *normal distribution* and is again illustrated in Fig. 3.1. The sampling distribution of the mean will be normal if the parent population is itself normally distributed, or if the population is not too markedly skewed and the sample is sufficiently large. Whilst these conditions are not always satisfied, the normal distribution is the most important distribution in sampling theory, and it is assumed for the remainder of this chapter that samples are drawn from a normal or near-normal population. Other sampling distributions are discussed in later chapters.

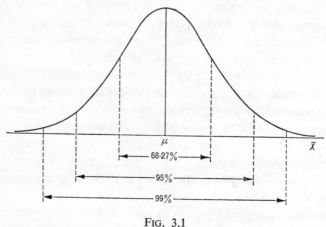

FIG. 3.1

In Fig. 3.1, the sample means ($\bar{X}$) are distributed in a symmetrical way (normally distributed) about the population mean μ. Although the parent population may be asymmetrical (skew) the means of samples drawn from that population will be normally distributed, subject to certain conditions, around the population mean.

All normal curves are of the same general shape and characteristics, but they vary with respect to height and 'spread'. For the moment, however, it is convenient to consider the general characteristics of a normal distribution. A normal distribution is divided into two halves by the ordinate erected above its mean value, as shown in Fig. 3.1. 50% of the observations lie above the arithmetic mean and 50% below. 68·27% of the observations lie within the range $\mu \pm$ one standard deviation. 95% of the observations lie within the range $\mu \pm 1.96$ standard deviations. 99% of the observations lie within the range $\mu \pm 2.58$ standard deviations (Fig. 3.1). These characteristics of a normal distribution are of fundamental importance in understanding the logic of tests of inference. If a variable is normally distributed then it may be stated with certainty that 95% of all the observations will fall within a certain range of the mean, that is, within 1.96 standard deviations in either a plus or minus direction. Equally it may be stated that 99% of the observations will fall within a certain range of the mean, that is, within 2.58 standard deviations in either a plus or minus direction. The range for 100% of the observations cannot be stated with any certainty but a range can be specified for any percentage of the observations less than this.*

These characteristics of a normal distribution may now be employed to make statements about the relationship between a population mean and the means of samples drawn from that population. For repeated random samples of size N drawn from a population, 95% of the sample means will lie, as mentioned, within a certain specified range of the population mean. This can be put in a different way, by stating that there is a 95% chance that any one sample mean will lie within the specified range. Expressed in this way the notion of probability is introduced. Thus there is a probability of 0.95 (95% chance) that any one sample mean ($\bar{X}$) will lie within the range $\mu \pm 1.96$ standard deviations. By extension there is a probability of 0.99 (99% chance) that $\bar{X}$ will lie within the range $\mu \pm 2.58$ standard deviations. There is a probability of 0.6827 (68.27% chance) that $\bar{X}$ will lie within the range $\mu \pm$ one standard deviation, and so on.

The results of the discussion so far may be summarized as follows: The means of repeated samples of size N drawn from a population with mean μ, will be normally distributed about the

---

* Another property of the normal distribution is that both tails of the curve continually approach, but never actually touch, the horizontal axis (abscissa). For this reason the range for 100% of the observations cannot be stated since mathematically the curve extends to infinity in both directions.

population mean. This is called the sampling distribution of the mean. By making use of the characteristics of a normal distribution the distribution of sample means about the population mean can be precisely determined. Specifically we can determine the probability that a single sample mean will lie within a certain range of values, or outside a certain range of values.

The basis of the discussion outlined at the beginning of this section may now be somewhat clearer to the reader. Before explaining this in greater detail one further characteristic of sampling distributions must be talked about. It was mentioned above that normal curves may vary with respect to their height and 'spread'. This is illustrated in Fig. 3.2, where two normal

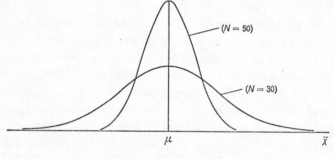

FIG. 3.2

(sampling) distributions are illustrated, both with the same mean μ. They differ with respect to height and 'spread'. In other words they vary in the extent to which the observations are dispersed around the mean μ.

What determines this dispersion? The two factors which determine the dispersion of sample means around the population mean are—(a) the *size of the sample,* and (b) the *standard deviation* of the population from which the samples are drawn. The larger the size of sample the more likely it is that the sample mean $(\bar{X})$ will approximate to the population mean (μ). To express it simply, large samples are 'more accurate'; a sample of 100 is likely to reflect more closely its parent population than a sample of, say, 25. Hence, if repeated samples of, say, 100 observations are taken, the sample means may be expected to be grouped fairly closely around the population mean.

The other factor which determines the distribution of sample means around the population mean is the standard deviation of the population (σ) from which the samples are drawn. If there is considerable variation in the population then the means of samples drawn from that population will also vary more than they would if the population values were grouped closely together. For example, there is considerable variation in the earnings of *all* adult workers in Ireland, and the means of random samples of, say, 50 workers may also vary quite markedly depending on the chance composition of each sample. There is much less variation in the earnings of all company directors in Ireland, and hence one would expect less variation in the mean earnings of random samples of 50 company directors.

Thus, the dispersion of sample means around the population mean is determined by the size of the samples and by the population standard deviation (σ). The dispersion of sample means around the population mean is described by a measure called the *standard error*. The standard error is calculated from the formula $\sigma/\sqrt{N}$, that is its value depends upon sample size and the standard deviation of the population from which the samples are drawn. The larger the sample and the smaller the standard deviation the smaller will be the standard error.*

In Fig. 3.2 above, repeated samples of size 50, and size 30 respectively, have been drawn from a population with a given mean μ, and standard deviation σ. The two sampling distributions though both of the same general shape vary with respect to height, and spread or dispersion. The dispersion of the sample means around the population mean is described by the standard deviation of the sample means—the standard error.

We are now in a position to describe more fully the relationship between population means and sample means. The means

* It is important to appreciate the distinction between the standard deviation of the parent population and the standard deviation of the distribution of sample means drawn from that population. The latter is referred to as the standard error.

of repeated samples of size N from a given population will be normally distributed around the population mean, with a standard error determined by the size of the samples and the standard deviation of the parent population. 95% of the sample means will be included in the range $\mu \pm 1.96$ standard errors, and 99% of the sample means will be included in the range $\mu \pm 2.58$ standard errors. There is a 95% chance, or a probability of 0.95, that any given sample mean will lie within the range $\mu \pm 1.96$ standard errors, and a probability of 0.99, or a 99% chance, that the sample mean will fall within the range $\mu \pm 2.58$ standard errors.

3.3   Tests of significance

The application of these theoretical principles to problems of estimation and hypothesis-testing will now be considered. Suppose first that it is desired to estimate the value of a population mean using the results of a sample. A random sample of a certain number of units is taken and the arithmetic mean $(\bar{X})$ is calculated. The sample mean $(\bar{X})$ is the best estimate available of the unknown population mean μ. However, since sample means drawn from a given population vary amongst themselves and from the population mean, it is desirable to qualify this estimate. It has been noted that in 95% of cases a sample mean $(\bar{X})$ will lie within the range ± 1.96 standard errors from the population mean. It also follows from this that in 95% of cases the population mean (μ) will lie within the range ± 1.96 standard errors from a given sample mean $(\bar{X})$, that is, the population mean (μ) will lie within the range $\bar{X} \pm 1.96$ standard errors. Hence, given the sample mean $(\bar{X})$ it is only necessary to calculate the standard error and then state 'the population mean lies within the range $\bar{X} \pm 1.96$ standard errors'. However, this statement must be qualified since it is in only 95% of cases that the statement will be true. It may be that the particular sample mean $(\bar{X})$ is one of the 5% of sample means which falls outside the range $\mu \pm 1.96$ standard errors. If this is so then the population mean will also lie outside the range $\bar{X} \pm 1.96$ standard errors. Since the population mean is unknown, we cannot be certain that any particular sample mean ($\bar{X}$) lies within the range $\mu \pm 1.96$ standard errors. Consequently, it is necessary to qualify the estimate of the population mean by stating 'it is 95% certain that the population mean lies within the range $\bar{X} \pm 1.96$ standard errors'. In 95 cases out of 100 we shall be correct in our estimate of the population mean, but in 5 cases out of 100 we shall be wrong. Alternatively, it could be stated that 'in 99% of cases (it is 99% certain that) the population mean will lie within the range $\bar{X} \pm 2.58$ standard errors'. *A priori* such a statement will be correct 99 times out of 100 and in this sense we can be 'more confident' that the population mean will lie within the range calculated. On the other hand it has been necessary to increase the interval within which the population mean is estimated to lie. The notions of 'confidence and 'confidence intervals' are further elaborated in Example 3.1.

EXAMPLE 3.1

A random sample of 100 Irishmen 21 years of age and over results in a mean height of 68 in. The standard deviation height of all Irishmen 21 years of age and over is known to be 2.5 in. Estimate the mean height of all Irishmen 21 years of age and over using the results of the sample. Here $\bar{X} = 68.0$ in., $\sigma = 2.5$ in., $N = 100$. It is required to estimate μ.

The 'best estimate' for μ is $\bar{X}$, i.e., 68.0 in. Generally, however, it will be desirable to express the estimate for μ in the form of an interval, within which it is reasonably certain that μ will fall. Means of samples of 100 Irishmen 21 years of age and over will be normally distributed around the unknown population mean (μ) with a standard error given by $\sigma/\sqrt{N}$, written $\sigma_{\bar{X}}$:

$$\sigma_{\bar{X}} = \sigma/\sqrt{N} = 2.5/\sqrt{100} = 2.5/10 = 0.25$$

In 95% of cases, a sample mean $\bar{X}$ will lie within the interval $\mu \pm 1.96\sigma_{\bar{X}}$, i.e., within the interval $\mu \pm 1.96 \times 0.25 = \mu \pm 0.49$. Conversely, in 95% of cases the population mean (μ) will lie within the interval $\bar{X} \pm 1.96\sigma_{\bar{X}} = \bar{X} \pm 0.49$.

Since $\bar{X} = 68.0$ in., the interval for the estimate of μ can be written 68.0 ± 0.49, i.e., 67.51–68.49 in. This estimate for μ will

be correct 95 times out of 100; in other words, we can be 95%
certain that this estimate for μ is correct. In 5% of cases we shall
be wrong and μ will lie outside the interval calculated. This
interval for the estimate of μ is called a *confidence interval* and in
the particular example above is referred to as a *95% confidence
interval*.

The 99% confidence interval for the estimate of μ may also be
calculated. This is given by $\bar{X} \pm 2{\cdot}58\sigma_{\bar{X}}$, i.e.

$$68{\cdot}0 \pm 2{\cdot}58 \times 0{\cdot}25 = 68{\cdot}0 \pm 0{\cdot}65,$$

or 67·35–68·65 in. Thus we can be 99% confident that μ lies
within the range 67·35–68·65 in. A comparison of the two con
fidence intervals shows that in the second case the estimate wil
be wrong only once in 100 times, instead of 5 times in 100; this
increased confidence has been achieved at the cost of widening
the possible interval for the estimate of μ.

Confidence intervals other than 95 and 99% may sometimes
be used. For example, the 90% confidence interval for μ above is
given by $\bar{X} \pm 1{\cdot}64\sigma_{\bar{X}}$, i.e. 67·59–68·41 in. (note that this confidence interval is narrower than the others, but the probability
of being incorrect is higher, 10 times in 100). However, the 95 and
99% confidence intervals are most commonly used. The limits
attached to the confidence interval are called *confidence limits*—
thus, the 95% confidence limits for μ in the example above are
67·51 and 68·49 in.

To summarize the results of the above example: Given that
the mean of a random sample of 100 Irishmen 21 years of age
and over is 68·0 in., and given that the population standard
deviation* is 2·5 in., we can be 95% confident that the mean
height of all Irishmen 21 years of age and over lies between 67·51
and 68·49 in., and 99% confident that the mean height lies
between 67·35 and 68·65 in.

* With respect to the example quoted concerning the estimate of the mean
height of Irishmen, 21 years of age and over, it may occur to the reader that
since the population mean (μ) is unknown it is likely that the population
standard deviation (σ) will also be unknown. This would generally be the
case. In this event the standard deviation (s) of the sample is used instead
to calculate the standard error—see Chapter 4.

The application of these principles of statistical inference to tests of hypotheses will now be explained. In problems of this kind the object is to determine whether a sample statistic and a population parameter are consistent with one another, or whether two or more sample results are consistent with one another. These tests are often referred to as *tests of significance*.

Suppose a sample of observations of a certain variable is taken and it is postulated that this sample has been drawn from a population with a certain mean; let us call this mean μ_O, and the standard deviation σ. The question may then arise— is the result of the sample consistent with the hypothesis that the sample has been drawn from a population with mean μ_O? In general, we would not expect the sample mean, $\bar{X}$, to be exactly equal to the population mean μ_O, but if the hypothesis were true we would expect the sample mean, $\bar{X}$, to be close to μ_O in value. In fact, if the hypothesis were true, we would expect that in 95 cases out of 100 the sample mean, $\bar{X}$, would lie in the interval $\mu_O \pm 1\cdot96\sigma_{\bar{X}}$ Suppose it is found that the sample mean, $\bar{X}$, does lie within the 95% confidence interval $\mu_O \pm 1\cdot96\sigma_{\bar{X}}$. In this case it may be concluded that the result of the sample is consistent with the hypothesis that the sample has been drawn from a population with mean μ_O; to express it more briefly the difference between $\bar{X}$ and μ_O is *not significant*.

Suppose, on the other hand, that the sample mean, $\bar{X}$, is found to lie outside the interval $\mu_O \pm 1\cdot96\sigma_{\bar{X}}$. One explanation for this is that, by chance, we have struck one of the 5 cases in 100 where the sample mean falls outside the 95% confidence interval. By its nature, however, this is unlikely. An alternative explanation is that the hypothesis is untrue—that the sample has *not* been drawn from a population with mean μ_O. By convention, this second explanation is always accepted. The sample mean, $\bar{X}$, and the population mean μ_O are said to be *significantly different*, and the hypothesis that the sample has been drawn from a population with mean μ_O is rejected. It is, of course, possible that the sample *has* been drawn from a population with mean μ_O, and that the sample mean in question is one which, by chance, falls outside the 95% confidence inter-

E

val, but the probability that this is so is very small—only 0·05. It is more reasonable to conclude that the sample in question was not drawn from a population with mean μ_0, that is the difference between the sample mean, $\bar{X}$, and the population mean μ_0 is *significant*. This may be illustrated by the hypothetical Example 3.2.

EXAMPLE 3.2

A motor manufacturing company claims for a new car model a petrol consumption of 45 m.p.g. with a standard deviation of 5 m.p.g. An independent test of 25 new cars by a consumer association results in a mean consumption of 42 m.p.g. Is this consistent with the company's claim?

Here $\mu_0 = 45\cdot0$, $\sigma = 5\cdot0$, $\bar{X} = 42\cdot0$, $N = 25$. The object of the test is to determine whether the sample mean value of 42·0 m.p.g. is consistent with the assumed population mean of 45·0 m.p.g.

If the company's claim is correct, repeated sample tests of 25 new cars should in 95% of cases result in a mean petrol consumption within the interval $\mu \pm 1\cdot96\sigma_{\bar{X}}$, where $\mu = 45\cdot0$.

$$\sigma_{\bar{X}} = \sigma/\sqrt{N} = 5/\sqrt{25} = 5/5 = 1$$

In 95% of cases the mean petrol consumption should lie within the interval $45\cdot0 \pm 1\cdot96 \times 1 = 45\cdot0 \pm 1\cdot96$, i.e., 43·04–46·96.

In this particular case, however, the sample mean of 42·0 m.p.g. falls outside the 95% confidence interval. Indeed, as the reader may verify, it also falls outside the 99% confidence interval. This means that if the hypothesis were true (if the company's claim were correct), we should expect to obtain a mean petrol consumption as low as 42·0 m.p.g. in rather less than one test in 100 just due to chance. Since this probability is so small, doubt is cast on the company's claim. We conclude that the difference between the sample mean and the assumed population mean is significant—we reject the hypothesis that the sample has been drawn from a population with mean $\mu_0 = 45\cdot0$. (The actual population mean is almost certainly less than 45·0.)

The example above illustrates the general procedure for tests of hypotheses. It is assumed that there is *no* significant difference between the population mean and the sample mean (or whatever may be the two figures which are compared); this is called the *null hypothesis*. The result of the test will either support or reject the null hypothesis—in the latter case the difference between the population parameter and the sample statistic is said to be significant. It should be noted that the interpretation of 'significant' depends to some extent upon the confidence interval used in the test. In the example above, if the mean petrol consumption for the sample had been 42·8 m.p.g. (instead of 42·0), this would have fallen outside the 95% confidence interval but inside the 99% confidence interval. Hence, if the 95% confidence interval had been used in the test the difference between μ_o (45·0) and $\bar{X}$ (42·8) would be significant, but if the 99% confidence interval were used the difference between μ_o and $\bar{X}$ would not be significant. This can be summarized by saying that the difference between μ_o and $\bar{X}$ *is significant at the 5% level but not significant at the 1% level.*

Finally, the result of such tests cannot be claimed to *prove* that the hypothesis is right or wrong. In the example above, although the difference between the sample mean ($\bar{X}$) and the population mean (μ_o) was regarded as significant it is possible that, by chance, the particular sample selected may be one of the 1% whose means lie outside the 99% interval. Conversely, if the sample mean was found to lie within the 95% confidence interval, this does not *prove* that the sample has been selected from a population with mean $\mu_o = 45·0$. All we can say is that the result of the test either supports or does not support the hypothesis. In other words the terms 'not significant' and 'significant' simply mean that the results obtained are respectively likely or unlikely to have occurred by chance.

It will be obvious to the reader that there is a relationship between significance and probability levels. By significance is meant that an observed result is unlikely to have arisen by chance; the result is considered to be a real difference and not due to sampling error. By convention the 5% (0·05 probability) level is taken as being significant. Such a result would occur by chance 5 times in 100, or once in 20 times. These, however, are long odds (19/1 against the result being due to chance) so the result is unlikely to have arisen by chance at a 5% level of significance. If the observed result has a probability of 0·02 (2% level of significance) it is more significant than a 5% level. A result at a 2% level of significance would occur by chance only once in 50 times. Stricter criteria can be taken such as a 1% (0·01 probability) level of significance; a result at this level would occur by chance once in 100 times. A result at a 0·1% (0·001 probability) level of significance would occur by chance once in 1000 times. If one sets out to adopt high levels of significance, the larger the sample required will be, and the more costly will be the experiments.

The examples quoted above are very simple examples of the application of the principles of statistical inference. It is hoped, however, that the methodology and terminology used may help the reader to grasp the general purpose and meaning of other tests of significance which will be discussed in the following chapters. Terms such as confidence intervals, confidence limits, significance and similar expressions will be referred to subsequently and the purpose of this chapter is to explain the meaning of these terms.

3.4   Selection of samples

The various methods by which sample data are collected have not yet been discussed and the foregoing discussion has been based on the assumption that simple random sampling has been used. In practice it is not always possible, or even desirable, to employ simple random sample designs and this section includes a brief discussion of some other types of sample design.

In setting up a sample survey the principal considerations are the type of sample design to be used and the size of the sample. It has already been explained that the larger the size of the sample the more closely the sample means will be dispersed around the population mean (μ), and so the smaller will be the 95%, and

99%, confidence limits for the mean. Let us assume that a sample mean is used to estimate the population mean. The larger the sample the smaller will be the estimated range, at the 95 and 99% levels, for the population mean. In selecting the sample therefore it is necessary to decide how precise one wishes the estimate to be. Against this must be balanced the increasing cost and time required for a larger sample.

Given the requirements of a study, methods are available for determining the minimum sample size required and the most efficient type of sample design to use, subject to constraints such as time and money. Both these problems involve complex technical matters which need not be discussed here. However, certain types of sample design which frequently arise in medical research will be outlined.

Reference has already been made to *simple random samples* and indeed the discussion in Sections 3.1–3.3 has been based on the concept of simple random sampling. This is the most basic type of sample design. In principle, a simple random sample is selected by numbering each unit in the population and then randomly selecting certain units from the population; the methods of random selection will not be described here but special tables have been compiled by mathematicians called random numbers which are commonly used for random selection and allocation. The method of selection ensures that each unit in the population has an equal chance of being selected in the sample.

A refinement of the simple random sample is the *stratified random sample*. The population is divided into groups, or strata, on the basis of certain characteristics, for example age and sex. A random sample is then selected from each stratum and the results for each stratum are combined to give the results for the total sample. The object of this type of sample design is to ensure that each stratum in the population is represented in the sample in certain fixed proportions which are determined in advance. For example if we wished to determine the smoking habits of the national population, obviously age and sex are important factors. We might wish to select a sample in which the age and sex composition of the sample would exactly reflect the age and sex composition of the whole population. With a simple random sample it is unlikely that the age and sex composition of the sample would *exactly* reflect these characteristics in the national population. However, by dividing the population for each sex into certain age-groups and selecting a random sample within each age-group for males *and* females, it can be ensured that the proportion of each age-group and each sex in the total sample will be identical with these proportions in the total population. Although in this example the sample proportions reflect exactly these proportions in the population, not all stratified random samples are selected in this way. Certain strata may be deliberately 'over-represented' in the sample, while others are 'under-represented'. The important point is that the sample proportions are pre-determined. For this reason stratified random samples are often preferred to simple random samples, and the sampling error in a stratified random sample is usually less than the sampling error in a simple random sample of the same size.

In medical research studies, the use of what are called *control groups* is a common and important technique of analysis. As an example, interest may be focused on a group of persons who suffer from coronary insufficiency. Data will be collected, concerning this group of persons, which are considered relevant to the inquiry, such as age, occupation, smoking history, and so on. We will then wish to determine whether or not any of these data are important or *significant* in relation to the condition being studied. For this purpose, it will generally be necessary to compare the group of patients with another group who do not suffer from coronary insufficiency, but who in other respects may be assumed to be comparable with the group of patients. The group who do not suffer from coronary insufficiency constitute the control group, and provide a basis of comparison with the group of patients. It might be found, for instance, that the mean serum cholesterol of the group of patients is 280 mg %. Obviously this result is of little value unless we can compare it with some standard. Is a mean cholesterol level of 280 mg % significantly higher than the mean serum cholesterol level for the whole population of which the group of patients are assumed to form a part? To test this hypothesis a suitable control group is selected and the mean serum cholesterol of the control group is calculated. It is then possible, using the kind of technique described in the previous section, to determine whether or not the mean for the control group is significantly different from the mean for the group of patients. If the two means *are* significantly different it is reasonable to suppose that raised serum cholesterol is an associated factor in coronary insufficiency.

In principle, the control group is randomly selected, with or without stratification, from the population under study, and is taken to be representative of that population. In practice, in medical studies the selection of control groups often presents difficulties and controls may have to be used which are not in fact randomly selected from the population, although for the purpose of the study it is assumed that the control group is suitably representative. For example, controls may be selected from amongst visitors to a particular hospital, employees of a particular organization, or persons who attend a certain clinic. Care must be exercised in using samples of this kind as control groups. It is important to specify beforehand the required characteristics of the control group, and to identify the particular population which the control group is taken to represent; is it to represent a particular social group, a particular age group, or a particular geographical area? The general purpose of control groups, however, is straightforward; they are designed as a basis for comparison by which appropriate tests of significance of factors related to the condition of interest, may be made.

A commonly used type of control group is the 'matched sample'; the control group and the original group of patients are identical with respect to certain characteristics such as age, sex, occupation, and so on. When a patient enters the study he is 'matched' with a control with the same characteristics. The two groups are then compared to see whether or not they differ significantly with regard to any other characteristics, for example serum cholesterol or obesity, which are suspected to be associated or causal factors. The aim here, of course, is to 'standardize' the two groups with respect to these characteristics.

Another type of sample design involves what is called a *'double-blind' trial* which is commonly used to assess the efficacy of a new treatment. It is called 'double-blind' because neither the patients nor the physician and his team know which 'treatment' a particular patient receives. Bias, for or against the new treatment, on the part of the physician and his team is then eliminated and patient bias is also prevented, which allows a more objective assessment. The 'treatment' a particular patient receives is known only during the course of the trial to a non-participant, generally a statistician. Let us suppose that it is required to test the efficacy of a new anti-hypertensive. The physician collects a group of patients with a defined type of hypertension. These patients are divided into two groups by random allocation; so the two groups should be very similar. There will then be a *treatment group*, the patients who receive the new anti-hypertensive, and a *control group*, the patients who receive a dummy tablet or placebo which is identical in appearance to the new anti-hypertensive. The placebo is important since it ensures that the two groups of patients remain uniform with regard to psychological effect. A 'double-blind' trial could also be designed to determine whether or not the new anti-hypertensive is as effective as an anti-hypertensive in everyday use. Then one group would receive the new drug and one group the old drug but otherwise the trial would remain the same. Differences between the groups are noted during the trial. At the conclusion of the study tests of significance will be applied to decide whether the observed differences are real (significant) or are likely to have occurred by chance (not significant).

In medical research literature references are often made to retrospective and prospective studies, and cross-sectional and longitudinal studies. In a *retrospective study* a group with a certain condition is taken and then one 'looks back' to elucidate the cause or causes. In a retrospective study of coronary heart disease a group of patients who had already suffered from this condition would be included, and then by history-taking, examination and investigation an effort is made to determine certain causative factors. A control group without coronary heart disease will be required for comparison.

A *prospective study* begins with a population in which the condition to be studied has not occurred. The population is followed forwards to determine the number of subjects developing the condition. In a prospective study of coronary heart disease a population without this condition is followed forwards and characteristics of those who later develop coronary heart disease are compared with those who do not. Those persons who do not develop the condition are the controls.

Retrospective and prospective studies have each distinct advantages and disadvantages in special circumstances. In retrospective studies great stress must be placed on memory and past history; in addition, bias of various kinds is common. On the other hand, a retrospective study is generally cheaper to carry out, takes a shorter time to conduct, and requires less staff than a prospective study. A retrospective study may be very useful for investigating a suspected association between two characteristics which ideally might be explored by a study of prospective type, for example the effects of virus infections during pregnancy.

A *cross-sectional study* could be described as an 'instant' study. Patients or subjects are examined for some particular characteristic or characteristics at one point in time. A cross-sectional study can also determine associations between a disease and a characteristic, for example type A hepatitis and raised serum glutamic oxaloacetic transaminase (SGOT). Certain types of hospital study may be cross-sectional in design and, of course, the national population census is also a good example of this type of survey.

A *longitudinal study* as its name suggests is a study which proceeds lengthwise, over a period of time, and can be associated with either a retrospective or a prospective study.

It is usual in many studies, but particularly those which involve high cost, to undertake a preliminary investigation using a small sample of the population to be studied. This investigation is called a *pilot study* and its purpose is to pinpoint unforeseen difficulties which may arise in the study proper, and to correct these difficulties before the main study begins.

This chapter has attempted to explain the basic ideas and

applications of statistical inference. The aim has been to enable the reader to grasp the purpose and interpretation of the many and varied applications of statistical inference without the need to understand the particular statistical techniques involved. In the following chapters examples of the application of these techniques will be illustrated and it is hoped that the reader will now be familiar with expressions such as confidence limits, standard errors, level of significance, controls, and so on. A great deal of the difficulty which arises in interpreting articles published in medical, social, and economic journals can be avoided by an understanding of certain elementary concepts and terminology used in statistical analysis, and it is hoped that this chapter has helped in clarifying these concepts.

4

4.1 Examples of estimation and tests of significance

The basic principles of statistical inference which were explained in the previous chapter will now be illustrated and developed by means of a number of examples. The examples included here cover a variety of the most common types of statistical tests which are used in medical research. Other types of tests will be described in a later chapter.

EXAMPLE 4.1

The weights of 100 medical students, randomly selected from amongst all medical students at a particular centre, are recorded. The population is assumed to be normally distributed with a standard deviation of 12·25 lb. The mean of the sample is $\bar{X} = 174·14$ lb, and the aim is to estimate the mean weight of all medical students at this centre. Hence given $\bar{X}$, the sample mean, it is required to estimate μ, the population mean.

In the previous chapter it was explained that if repeated samples of size N are drawn from a normal population the sample means will be normally distributed around the population mean with a standard error of $\sigma/\sqrt{N} = \sigma_{\bar{X}}$. It was further stated that 95% of all sample means will lie within the range of $\mu \pm 1·96\sigma_{\bar{X}}$ (the 95% confidence interval) and 99% of all sample means will lie within the range $\mu \pm 2·58\sigma_{\bar{X}}$ (the 99% confidence interval). It follows from this that in 95% of cases the population mean (μ) will lie within the range $\bar{X} \pm 1·96\sigma_{\bar{X}}$, and that in 99% of cases μ will lie within the range $\bar{X} \pm 2·58\sigma_{\bar{X}}$ for any given sample mean ($\bar{X}$).

These properties may now be applied to estimate the mean weight of all medical students in the centre. Given $\bar{X} = 174·14$, the 95% confidence interval for μ is $174.14 \pm 1.96\sigma_{\bar{X}}$, where $\sigma_{\bar{X}} = \sigma/\sqrt{N}$. Given $\sigma = 12.25$ and $N = 100$, the standard error can be calculated as $\sigma/\sqrt{N} = 12.25/\sqrt{100} = 1.23$. The 95% confidence limits for μ are now $174.14 \pm 1.96 \times 1.23$, which gives the range 171.73 to 176.55 lb. Similarly, the 99% confidence limits for μ are given by

$$\bar{X} \pm 2.58\sigma_{\bar{X}} = 174.14 \pm 2.58 \times 1.23,$$

and the range then is 170.97 to 177.31 lb. On the basis of the sample we can be 95% confident that the mean weight of all medical students in the centre lies in the range 171.73 to 176.55 lb, and 99% confident that the mean weight of these students is in the range 170.97 to 177.31 lb.

At this stage several important points should be noted. First, the validity of an estimate of this kind depends upon the assumption that the means of repeated samples are normally distributed about the population mean. As we shall see later, not all sampling distributions are normal, and estimation procedures and tests of hypotheses based on the normal distribution should not be applied unless it can be reasonably assumed that the particular sampling distribution *is* normal. However, the normal distribution is the most important sampling distribution as well as being the most useful for purposes of exposition. The techniques described here and in the previous chapter, based on the characteristics of the normal distribution, are applied in a similar way to other sampling distributions.

Secondly, in cases where the population is finite, as in the example above, the 95 and 99% confidence intervals will be somewhat less than stated (that is, $\pm 1.96\sigma_{\bar{X}}$ and $\pm 2.58\sigma_{\bar{X}}$ respectively). However, unless the sample is quite large in relation to the population, this point may be ignored.

Thirdly, constant reference is made to 95 and 99% confidence limits, and the 95 and 99% confidence intervals, which represent the ranges between these limits. Any other confidence limits or intervals may be used; for example, in a normal distribution, 95.46% of all sample means fall within the limits $\mu \pm 2.0$ standard errors, 98% of all sample means fall within the limits $\mu \pm 2.33$

standard errors, 80% of all sample means fall within the limits $\mu \pm 1.28$ standard errors, and so on. Tables may be consulted to determine the range for any given percentage of sample means. However, the 95 and 99% confidence intervals are the ones most commonly used, though the 90, 98, and 99.9% confidence intervals are also used. For applied work, confidence intervals less than 95% (and certainly less than 90%) are seldom used.

The application of examples of this kind to medical research will be readily appreciated. It is often desired to determine some characteristic of a population such as height or blood pressure, and seldom possible to examine every unit in that population. By making use of the characteristics of the normal distribution as explained above, population values can be estimated from the results of a sample. The confidence interval for the estimate of μ may, of course, be reduced by increasing the size of the sample, since the standard error decreases as the sample size increases.

EXAMPLE 4.2

A random sample of 100 males has a mean age of 40 years. Could this have been drawn from a population whose ages are normally distributed around a mean of 35 years and a standard deviation of 15 years?

Here the object is to determine whether or not a sample mean ($\bar{X}$) and a population mean (μ) are significantly different. We set up the hypothesis that the sample mean and the population mean are not significantly different; that the sample has been drawn from a population with mean μ, and that μ and $\bar{X}$ differ only by chance. This is the null hypothesis, which is accepted or rejected depending on the result of the test.

If repeated samples of 100 are drawn from a population with a mean of 35·0 and a standard deviation of 15·0, the means of these samples will be normally distributed about a mean of 35·0 with a standard error of $\sigma/\sqrt{N} = 15/\sqrt{100} = 1.5$. Further, 95% of all sample means will lie within the range $35.0 \pm 1.96 \times 1.5$, and 99% of all sample means will lie within the range $35.0 \pm 2.58 \times 1.5$. These ranges are 32·06 to 37·94, and 31·13 to 38·87 respectively. The sample mean ($\bar{X} = 40.0$) lies outside the 99% confidence interval, and of course the 95% interval. If the hypothesis were true, there would be a less than 1% chance of obtaining a random sample with a mean as different from μ as the one obtained. In 99% of cases we should expect the sample mean to lie within the range 31·13 to 38·87 years. Either we have struck a fluke or the hypothesis is untrue. Since the former is unlikely, we conclude that the hypothesis is untrue; the null hypothesis is rejected. The sample mean ($\bar{X}$) and the population mean (μ) are significantly different; the sample could not have been drawn from a population with a mean of 35 years. As a corollary, we may conclude that the sample has been drawn from a population with a mean greater than 35·0.

Applications similar to this are of great importance in medical research. It is frequently necessary to compare samples and populations in respect of certain variables such as age, weight, smoking experience, cholesterol, and so on. Thus, it is possible to establish whether or not a group of patients in a sample are older, heavier, smoke more, or have higher cholesterol levels than the population of which they are assumed to form a part. Tests of this kind involve a comparison between a sample statistic and a population parameter.

In Example 4.2, the population mean was known and the test of significance involved a comparison of the sample mean and the population mean. In most practical problems, however, the population parameter is unknown, and it is necessary to use what is called a control group. The use of a control group for this purpose was explained in the previous chapter (Section 3.4) and is shown in Example 4.3.

One of the aims of this study was to determine whether or not the mean cholesterol level of women of different age groups using oral contraceptives (the test group) was different from the mean serum cholesterol level of the general population of women of different age groups. Within each age group, the test group was compared with a control group, which was taken to represent the general population of women in that age group. From the table it will be seen that the mean cholesterol level for the test group exceeds the mean level for the control group in both age groups.

EXAMPLE 4.3

Mean values of serum-lipids in control and test groups

Mean serum-cholesterol (mg/100ml)							
Women aged 20–29				Women aged 30–39			
(1)	(2)			(3)	(4)		
Controls	Test group	(2)–(1)	P	Controls	Test group	(4)–(3)	P
181	198	17	<0·02	196	207	11	N.S.

N.S. = Not significant

Reprinted from the *Lancet.* Wynn V., Doar J. W. H., and Mills G. L. (1966), **2**, 720. Some effects of oral contraceptives on serum-lipid and lipoprotein levels. (Table abbreviated.) (By permission of the Authors, Editor, and Publishers.)

The question to be determined is whether or not the mean levels differ significantly, taking each group separately.

The method used for this type of test is very similar to that used to test the difference between a sample mean and a population mean. Suppose two random samples, of size N_1 and N_2 respectively, are drawn from the same (normal) population or from two normal distributions with identical means. The means of these two samples will probably be different just due to chance. Repeated pairs of random samples of size N_1 and N_2 will generate a whole series of differences between sample means (*sample mean differences*) which can be formed into a sampling distribution. In some cases the differences between the sample means will be zero, but in most cases there will be a difference between the sample means, just due to chance. The numerical magnitude of the sample mean differences will depend upon the standard deviation of the population from which the samples are drawn, and the size of each sample.*

* The sample mean differences will be distributed around a mean of zero with a standard error determined by the standard deviation of the parent population and the size of the two samples. The greater the standard deviation of the parent population the greater will be the probable variation between any two sample means. Conversely, the larger size of the two

In the same way that confidence limits can be established to determine whether or not a sample mean and a population mean are significantly different, confidence limits can also be calculated to determine whether or not two sample means differ significantly from one another. If repeated pairs of samples of size N_1 and N_2 are drawn from a population, it can be established that in 95% of cases the difference between the two sample means, written $\bar{X}_1 - \bar{X}_2$, will not exceed a certain numerical value, say $\pm d$. Similarly, it can be established that in 99% of cases the difference between $\bar{X}_1$ and $\bar{X}_2$ will not exceed a certain numerical value, say $\pm h$. Conversely, in 5% of cases the difference $\bar{X}_1 - \bar{X}_2$ will fall outside the limits $\pm d$, and in 1% of cases outside the limits $\pm h$.

Now suppose two random samples of size N_1 and N_2 are taken and the difference $\bar{X}_1 - \bar{X}_2$ is found to be outside the 95% confidence interval which has been calculated. Either we have struck a fluke, or the *two samples have not been drawn from the same population* (or from populations with identical means). If the two samples had been drawn from the same population we should not expect to obtain a difference between the two sample means as large as the one obtained. The null hypothesis, that the two samples have been drawn from the same population, or identical populations, is rejected.

This type of test proceeds as follows. The samples of size N_1 and N_2 are taken and the two sample means $\bar{X}_1$ and $\bar{X}_2$ calculated. The null hypothesis is applied. This asserts that the two samples have been drawn from the same population, or from populations with identical means, and that the difference between the two sample means is simply due to chance, i.e. is not significant. To test the null hypothesis the 95% and/or the 99% confidence limits for $\bar{X}_1 - \bar{X}_2$ are calculated. The precise methods by which these are calculated will not be explained here, but they are similar to those already explained to calculate the confidence limits for a sample mean. Suppose the 99% confidence limits are calculated and found to be $\pm l$. This means that, if the hypothesis is true, and if repeated pairs of samples of size N_1

samples the more likely it is that the two sample means will be relatively close in value. It is not necessary that the two samples be of equal size.

and N_2 are taken, in 99% of cases the difference between the two sample means $(\bar{X}_1 - \bar{X}_2)$ will not exceed $\pm l$. If for the two samples taken, it is found that $|\bar{X}_1 - \bar{X}_2| > l$, then either we have struck a fluke or the hypothesis is untrue.* Since the former event is unlikely, less than 1% chance, we reject the null hypothesis and conclude that the two sample means are significantly different. The two samples have not been drawn from the same population, or identical populations.

Let us now return to the example quoted, first considering the data for the 20–29 age group. The control group represents a sample of women from the general population of women aged 20–29. The test group represents a sample of women from the population of women aged 20–29 who use oral contraceptives. The mean cholesterol level for the control group can be written $\bar{X}_1 = 181$, and the mean cholesterol level for the test group as $\bar{X}_2 = 198$. The difference between the two sample means $|\bar{X}_1 - \bar{X}_2| = 17$. Now if the test group and the control group have been drawn from the same population, or two populations which are identical with respect to cholesterol levels, it is reasonable to expect that $\bar{X}_1$ and $\bar{X}_2$ will not be significantly different. Therefore it is desired to establish whether or not the difference (17) between the mean levels of the two groups is significant. The actual arithmetic of this example will not be shown here, but let us assume that the 95% confidence limits for $\bar{X}_1 - \bar{X}_2$ are calculated and found to be ±15. This means if the null hypothesis were true, that in 95% of cases the difference $|\bar{X}_1 - \bar{X}_2|$ would be 15 or less. The particular difference noted (17) exceeds this, and hence it is concluded that the difference between $\bar{X}_1$ and $\bar{X}_2$ is significant at the 5% level. At the 5% level of significance the null hypothesis is rejected.† This may be interpreted to mean that the control

* $|\bar{X}_1 - \bar{X}_2|$ means that the algebraic sign of the difference $\bar{X}_1 - \bar{X}_2$ is ignored.

† However, in this particular example the difference between the two means is not significant at the 1% level. The difference (17) falls *within* the 99% confidence interval. Thus, the probability of obtaining a difference between the two sample means of 17 or greater, if the hypothesis were true, is >0.01 but <0.05. It can also be shown that the difference falls *outside* the 98% confidence interval; the difference is significant at the 2% level. The

F

group and the test group have not been drawn from populations which are identical with respect to cholesterol levels. The test group differs significantly from the control group with respect to mean cholesterol level.

Consider now the 30–39 age group. $\bar{X}_1 = 196$ and $\bar{X}_2 = 207$, so that $|\bar{X}_1 - \bar{X}_2| = 11$. Again the null hypothesis that $\bar{X}_1$ and $\bar{X}_2$ differ only by chance is asserted, and this hypothesis is tested by calculating the 95 and 99% confidence limits for $\bar{X}_1 - \bar{X}_2$. Suppose that the 95% confidence limits are found to be ± 14. If the hypothesis were true then in 95% of cases the difference $|\bar{X}_1 - \bar{X}_2|$ would be 14 or less. The particular difference noted (11) falls within the 95% confidence interval and is consistent with the null hypothesis. The difference between the two means is not significant. This is denoted by the term 'N.S.' in the table; alternatively we could write '$P > 0.05$'. There is no evidence that the test group differs from the control group with respect to mean cholesterol level.

One further point may be noted here. Often, depending on the particular problem being studied, the mean and standard deviation of the control group may be used as estimates of the mean (μ) and standard deviation (σ) of the population, and the test conducted in exactly the same way as described in Example 4.2.

Example 4.4 illustrates another application of the type of test described in Example 4.3. The time between onset of symptoms and start of treatment is recorded for a propranolol-treated group of patients, and a control group who were given 'dummy' tablets or placebos. The mean time for the propranolol group is 16·2 hours with a standard error of 2·1 hr (S.E.M. = standard error of the mean). The mean time for the placebo group is 13·4 hours with a standard error of 1·4 hr. Then, $\bar{X}_1 = 16\cdot2$, $\bar{X}_2 = 13\cdot4$ and $|\bar{X}_1 - \bar{X}_2| = 2\cdot8$. Is this difference significant?

The null hypothesis maintains that the difference between the two means arises only by chance, and that the two groups have been drawn from populations which are identical with respect to

probability of obtaining a difference between the two sample means of 17 or more, if the hypothesis were true, is $<0\cdot02$. This is the meaning of the term '$P < 0\cdot02$' in the fourth column of the table.

EXAMPLE 4.4

Time between onset of symptoms and start of
treatment

Hours	No. of patients on:	
	Propranolol	Placebo
0–6	23	29
7–12	29	24
13–18	16	10
19–24	15	16
Over 24	8	4
Average time (hr)	*16·2*	*13·4*
±S.E.M.	*2·1*	*1·4*

Reprinted from the *Lancet*. Stephen S. A., *et al.* (1966), **2**, 1435.
Propanolol in acute myocardial infarction: A multicentre trial.
(By permission of the Authors, Editor, and Publishers.)

the time elapsing between onset of symptoms and start of treatment. The 95% confidence limits for $\bar{X}_1 - \bar{X}_2$ are calculated, and compared with the difference of 2·8 noted. In this particular example it is found that the difference between the two means is not significant; the difference of 2·8 falls within the 95% confidence limits. The null hypothesis is accepted; the time of onset of symptoms and start of treatment for the propranolol and placebo groups is not significantly different.

Both Examples 4.3 and 4.4 involve a comparison between a test group and some form of control group. It is the test group which is of particular interest, while the control group is used as a basis for comparison. The real interest is in whether or not the characteristics of the test group are consistent with the general population of which the test group is assumed to form a part, and the control group is taken to be representative of that population. Tests of this kind are frequently used in medical research, in particular to test the effects of new drugs or methods of treatment or to identify ways in which a particular group of persons differ from the general population.

EXAMPLE 4.5

Blood groups: lesion size

Lesion size (sq cm)	Blood groups A	Blood groups O
<0·5	66	87
0·5 but less than 1·0	52	90
1·0 but less than 1·5	66	90
1·5 but less than 2·0	16	17
2·0 but less than 2·5	22	14
2·5 but less than 3·0	2	4
3·0 but less than 3·5	1	3
3·5 but less than 4·0	0	3
Total	225	308
$\bar{X}$	0·996	0·957

Reprinted from the *Journal of Medical Genetics*. Bourke G. J., Clarke N., Thornton E. H. (1965), **2**, 122. Smallpox vaccination: ABO and rhesus blood groups. (Table abbreviated.) (By permission of the Authors, Editor, and Publishers.)

A variation of this type of test is where a comparison is made between two groups, neither of which is a control group. An example of this kind of test will now be explained.

The object in this example is to determine whether or not lesion size following smallpox vaccination varies between individuals of blood group A and individuals of blood group O. The mean lesion size for blood group A can be written $\bar{X}_1 = 0.996$ and for blood group O, $\bar{X}_2 = 0.957$. The difference

$$| \bar{X}_1 - \bar{X}_2 | = 0.039.$$

The null hypothesis asserts that this difference arises only by chance and that the two groups have been drawn from the same population, or from identical populations, with respect to lesion size. If the results of the test support the null hypothesis then it may be concluded that lesion size is independent of blood group, for the two blood groups concerned.

The 95% confidence limits for $\bar{X}_1 - \bar{X}_2$ are calculated as before; suppose these are found to be ± 0.102. With repeated sampling in 95% of cases $\bar{X}_1 - \bar{X}_2$ would lie between -0.102 and $+0.102$, if the hypothesis were true. The actual difference noted is 0.039. This falls within the 95% confidence interval and so the null hypothesis is accepted. The difference between the two sample means is not significant, and supports the hypothesis that lesion size is independent of blood group, for the two blood groups in the example.

Example 4.6 also involves a comparison of lesion size, following smallpox vaccination, between two sample groups. The means of the two groups can be written $\bar{X}_1 = 0.72$, $\bar{X}_2 = 1.15$ (shown as $\bar{X}_W$ and $\bar{X}_I$ respectively in the table). Hence, $|\bar{X}_1 - \bar{X}_2|$ equals 0.43. Is the difference between the two means significant? Again, the null hypothesis is set up, that the two groups have been drawn from populations which are identical with respect to lesion size. The 95% confidence interval for $\bar{X}_1 - \bar{X}_2$ is calculated. Suppose this is found to be -0.090 to $+0.090$.* If the hypothesis were true, in 95% of cases we should expect the difference between the two sample means to be $\leqslant$ (equal to or less than) 0.090. The actual difference noted (0.43) greatly exceeds this and the difference between the two sample means is significant at the 5% level. By calculating the 99 and 99.9% confidence intervals, it can also be shown that the difference is significant at the 1 and 0.1% levels. The null hypothesis, that the two samples have been drawn from identical populations with regard to lesion size following smallpox vaccination is rejected. It is concluded that lesion size is significantly greater among subjects who were 'ill'.

* The symbol '$\sigma(\bar{X}_W - \bar{X}_I)$' will be observed in the bottom right hand corner of the table. This is called the *standard error of the difference between sample means* and corresponds to the standard of error of the mean ($\sigma_{\bar{X}}$) already referred to in describing the sampling distribution of the mean. Like the standard error of the mean, it is used to calculate the confidence limits for the distribution of $\bar{X}_1 - \bar{X}_2$.

EXAMPLE 4.6

Lesion size

	0·00–0·49 sq cm	0·50–0·99 sq cm	1·0–1·49 sq cm	1·5–1·99 sq cm	2·0–2·49 sq cm	2·5 sq cm and over	Total	
Well	129 (62·0%)	109 (52·4%)	54 (26·3%)	11 (25·0%)	8 (17·0%)	3 (12·5%)	314 (42·7%)	$\bar{X}_W = 0·72$ sq cm
III	79 (38·0%)	99 (47·6%)	151 (73·7%)	33 (75·0%)	39 (83·0%)	21 (87·5%)	422 (57·3%)	$\bar{X}_I = 1·15$ sq cm
	208 (100%)	208 (100%)	205 (100%)	44 (100%)	47 (100%)	24 (100%)	736 (100%)	$\sigma(\bar{X}_W - \bar{X}_I) = 0·045$

Reprinted from the *Irish Journal of Medical Science*, Bourke G. J., and Clarke N. (1964), 6th Series, No. 458, 75. Some observations on clinical reactions following smallpox vaccinations. (By permission of the Authors and Editor.)

4.2   Student's *t* distribution

The examples discussed in the preceding section, and in Chapter 3, have been based on the properties of the normal distribution. We have assumed a normal distribution for the sampling distribution of the mean. This will be true provided the population from which the sample is drawn is itself normally distributed.

If the population is not normally distributed, or its distribution is unknown, it cannot be assumed that the distribution of sample means is normal, and the tests described are not strictly valid. Since in practice many populations are non-normal, or their distribution is unknown, this might appear to severely limit the application of tests based on the normal distribution.

However, for large samples (say greater than 50), it can generally be assumed that sample means are normally distributed, even if the populations from which they are drawn are non-normal. For samples of 100 or more, the sampling distribution of the mean can be assumed normal unless the population distribution is very markedly skewed. This is an important result since it greatly increases the range of application of tests based on the normal distribution.

Secondly, it will be recalled that the distribution of sample means involves the calculation of the standard error, defined as $\sigma_{\bar{X}} = \sigma/\sqrt{N}$, where σ is the population standard deviation. However, in most problems the population standard deviation is unknown, and the *sample* standard deviation (denoted by s) is used instead, as an estimate of the population standard deviation. In such cases the standard error is written $s_{\bar{X}} = s/\sqrt{N}$ or $\sigma_{\bar{X}} = \tilde{\sigma}/\sqrt{N}$, which denotes that the sample statistic has been used instead of the population parameter.

Unfortunately, the use of $s_{\bar{X}}$ rather than $\sigma_{\bar{X}}$ vitiates the use of the normal distribution in problems of estimation and tests of significance. Instead, it is necessary to make use of a sampling distribution called *Student's t distribution*, or simply the *t* distribution. This affects the tests of significance described above in one important respect; the confidence limits for the distribution of sample means around the population mean must be extended. Thus, using the normal distribution the 95% confidence limits for $\bar{X}$ are $\mu \pm 1 \cdot 96\sigma_{\bar{X}}$; with repeated random sampling 95% of sample means would lie within the range $\mu \pm 1 \cdot 96\sigma_{\bar{X}}$. Using the t distribution, the 95% confidence limits will be wider; how much wider depends upon the size of the sample. For samples of size 15, for example, the 95% confidence limits are given by $\mu \pm 2 \cdot 14s_{\bar{X}}$; with repeated random samples of size $N = 15$, 95% of sample means would fall within the interval $\mu - 2 \cdot 14s_{\bar{X}}$ to $\mu + 2 \cdot 14s_{\bar{X}}$. For samples of size 30, the 95% confidence limits are given by $\mu \pm 2 \cdot 04s_{\bar{X}}$. The smaller the sample the wider the confidence limits.

Student's t distribution is a symmetrical distribution similar in shape to the normal distribution and in fact it approaches the normal distribution as N, the sample size, increases.

Consider now Example 4.7. At first sight this example appears to be a variation of Examples 4.5 and 4.6. A group of 15 patients are given Atromid-S and the mean cholesterol level each month is compared with the initial cholesterol level of 228. After 1 month the mean cholesterol level is 190 and this is compared with the initial level; with $\bar{X}_1 = 228$ and $\bar{X}_2 = 190$ this gives $|\bar{X}_1 - \bar{X}_2| = 38$. This difference is then tested for significance as before. After 2 months the mean cholesterol level has fallen to 170 and this is also compared with the initial level, giving $|\bar{X}_1 - \bar{X}_3| = 58$, and so on. Altogether five tests of significance are involved.

However, Example 4.7 illustrates both qualifications discussed above. It is a small sample drawn from a population with unknown standard deviation. To employ the kinds of significance tests described it has to be assumed that the population (serum cholesterol levels) is normally distributed, or nearly so. Secondly, since the sample standard deviations have been used to compute standard errors it is necessary to use the properties of the t distribution rather than the normal distribution.

Working through the example, it is desired to determine whether or not the difference between the initial cholesterol level of 228 and the level after 1 month is significant. With $\bar{X}_1 = 228$, $\bar{X}_2 = 190$, the difference $\bar{X}_1 - \bar{X}_2| = 38$. As before, the 95% and/or 99% confidence limits for $\bar{X}_1 - \bar{X}_2$ are calculated; how-

EXAMPLE 4.7

Serum cholesterol changes in 15 patients taking Atromid-S (mg/100ml)

Case no.	Initial level	Trial period (months)				
		1	2	3	6	9
1	205	225	205	190	200	190
2	175	165	160	155	175	185
3	235	190	150	225	—	210
4	170	170	145	140	185	190
5	185	135	130	—	170	160
6	255	145	145	155	155	180
7	245	215	175	170	155	200
8	185	160	190	200	225	230
9	260	190	195	—	205	225
10	265	270	160	195	200	200
11	280	195	150	145	190	165
12	150	145	130	145	140	—
13	260	250	Died			
14	250	215	220	220	230	—
15	300	185	220	210	175	—
Mean	228	190	170	179	180	194
Mean change		−38	−58	−49	−48	−34
S.E.		±9·25	±10·99	±13·07	±14·41	±10·75
t		4·11	5·28	3·75	3·33	3·16
P		<0·01	<0·001	<0·01	<0·01	<0·02

Reprinted from the *British Medical Journal*, Goodhart J. M., and Dewar H. A. (1966), **1**, 325. Effect of Atromid-S on fibrinolytic activity in patients with ischaemic heart disease and normal blood cholesterol levels. (By permission of the Authors, Editor, and Publishers.)

ever, since the sample consists of only 15 persons we are dealing with a t distribution and the confidence limits will be somewhat wider than would be the case of a normal distribution. Having calculated the confidence limits it can then be determined whether or not the sample mean difference of 38 is significant. In this particular case the 99% confidence interval for $\bar{X}_1 - \bar{X}_2$ is approximately -28 to $+28$. The actual difference noted (38) falls outside this range and hence it is concluded that there is a significant difference between $\bar{X}_1$ and $\bar{X}_2$. Similarly, it may be shown that for each month of the trial the difference between the mean cholesterol level in that month and the initial mean level is significant. Similar methods are used for this test as for the two previous examples; the only difference is that because of the small sample, wider confidence limits must be used.

In the table of Example 4.7, the last lines show the calculations which arise in conducting the tests of significance. The fourth last line records the difference between the initial mean cholesterol level and the mean level in each subsequent month. The third last line records the standard error (S.E.).

In the second last line the values of t, the t of Student's t distribution, are obtained by dividing the 'mean change' $|\bar{X}_1 - \bar{X}_2|$ in line one by the standard error in line two. Thus, $|-38|/9{\cdot}25 = 4{\cdot}11$, $|-58|/10{\cdot}99 = 5{\cdot}28$, and so on.

A table of Student's t distribution is now consulted to determine whether the value of t is significant at the 1 or 5% level. With the normal distribution a value of $|\bar{X}_1 - \bar{X}_2|/\sigma_{\bar{X}}$ in excess of $1{\cdot}96$ would be significant at the 5% level, and a value in excess of $2{\cdot}58$ would be significant at the 1% level. With Student's t distribution, the 95 and 99% confidence limits are wider and the 'critical values' of t are consequently greater. However, in each case the values of t recorded in Example 4.7 are significant at the 5% level and in all cases except one at the 1% level. A value of t in excess of the 95% critical value signifies that the difference between the sample means falls outside the 95% confidence interval calculated. The critical values for t depend upon the size of the sample and the confidence limits used.

This brings us to the last line of the table which records various values for P (probability). The first value recorded, $P < 0{\cdot}01$, can be interpreted as follows: If the null hypothesis were true, a difference between the initial cholesterol level and the level after 1 month as large as the difference observed (38) would be expected to arise in less than one case in 100, just due to chance. Hence, the result has either occurred by chance or the hypothesis is untrue and there *is* a significant difference between the two means. By convention, the second alternative is accepted, and the null hypothesis is rejected. We conclude that Atromid-S has a significant effect upon cholesterol level within the period of the trial.

The values of P recorded indicate the level of significance of the difference between the two means. Where $P < 0.01$ the difference is significant at the 1 % level. Where $P < 0.001$, the difference is significant at the 0.1 % level. In the last case, $P < 0.02$ and this means that the difference is significant at the 2 % level but not at the 1 % level.

4.3 χ^2 distribution

Another important probability distribution which is widely used in medical statistics is the χ^2 (chi-square) distribution. Examples of the χ^2 distribution will now be discussed.

EXAMPLE 4.8

Technique of vaccination

	Scratch	Multiple-pressure	Total
Successful	372 (76·7%)	436 (85·7%)	808 (81·3%)
Unsuccessful	113 (23·3%)	73 (14·3%)	186 (18·7%)
Total	485 (100%)	509 (100%)	994 (100%)

$$\chi^2 = 13 \cdot 10; \; n = 1; \; P < 0 \cdot 001$$

Reprinted from the *British Medical Journal*. Bourke G. J., and Clarke N. (1963), **2**, 281. Smallpox vaccination: Success rates of scratch and multiple-pressure techniques. (By permission of the Authors, Editor, and Publishers.)

In this example the data are presented in a form known as a contingency table involving a bi-variate classification. Data are classified by technique of vaccination and by whether or not the vaccination was successful.

The problem here is to determine whether or not there is any significant difference in the success rates of the two methods of vaccination. The success rate is 76·7% for the scratch technique and 85·7% for the multiple-pressure technique. Is this difference just due to chance or is the success rate significantly higher when the multiple-pressure technique is used? It will be noticed that this problem is similar in principle to the tests of significance already discussed.

To answer this question, the null hypothesis that there is no difference between the success rates of the two techniques is used and then what are called 'expected' frequencies are calculated for each cell (compartment), excluding the total column and total row, within the table. The actual method of computation of these expected' frequencies need not detain us here. *They are the frequencies to be expected if there were no differences between the two techniques.* The actual or 'observed' frequencies and the 'expected' frequencies are then compared. If the observed and expected frequencies in each cell are the same then it is concluded that there is no difference in the success rates of the two techniques and the null hypothesis would be accepted. In practice, the observed and expected frequencies are almost certain to vary to some degree.* Some method must be established to decide whether or not the differences between the observed and expected frequencies are just due to chance or arise because of a significant difference in the success rates of the two techniques. It will be observed that this line of reasoning is very similar to that used to determine whether or not a sample mean and a population mean are significantly different.

The method used to determine whether or not the observed and expected frequencies are significantly different is quite simple. The observed and expected frequencies in each cell are compared, and from these comparisons a measure called χ^2 (which is a

---

* In the same way that if an unbiased coin is tossed 100 times, the 'expected' number of heads is 50; in practice the number of heads is unlikely to be *exactly* 50. However, if heads turned up 75 times, we might well be suspicious, since on *a priori* grounds the probability of this occurring by chance seems small.

number) is derived. In general terms χ^2 is a measure of the overall difference between the observed and expected frequencies. If the observed and expected frequencies in each cell are equal, the value of χ^2 will be zero; the greater the *relative* differences between the observed and expected frequencies the greater the value of χ^2.

When the value of χ^2 has been calculated a statistical table of the χ^2 distribution may be consulted to determine whether or not the value of χ^2 obtained is significant at the 5 or 1 % level, or indeed any other level. The greater the value of χ^2 the more likely it is that the difference between the observed and expected frequencies is significant. This may be interpreted to mean that a value of χ^2 as large as the one obtained is unlikely to have arisen by chance.

One further point may be mentioned. It may have occurred to the reader that the more cells there are in the table, the greater the number of comparisons between observed and expected frequencies, and the larger will be the value of χ^2 (χ^2 is always equal to or greater than 0). This is quite correct. Hence, whether the difference between the observed and expected frequencies is significant or not depends not only on the value of χ^2 but also on the number of independent comparisons between observed and expected frequencies. The number of independent comparisons involved in any χ^2 test is called the *number of degrees of freedom*, frequently denoted by *n* or by the initials *d.f.* Thus, having calculated the value of χ^2, the table of χ^2 distribution is consulted to find whether the value of χ^2 obtained is significant or not given the number of degrees of freedom in that particular test.

Returning now to Example 4.8, at the bottom of the table the value of χ^2 is given as 13·10. The figures in the table are the observed frequencies; the expected frequencies which have to be calculated to obtain χ^2 are omitted from the table. The number of degrees of freedom in the example is one ($n = 1$). This may seem odd since the number of cells in the table is four (excluding the marginal totals recorded in the last row and column) implying four comparisons between observed and expected frequencies. However, there is only one *independent* comparison in the sense that given the marginal totals, once one cell is filled in the other three frequencies are automatically determined. Consulting the table of the χ^2 distribution it is found that the value of χ^2 at the 1% level of significance with $n = 1$, is 6·64. This means that, if the null hypothesis were true that there was no difference between the success rates of the two techniques, in 99% of cases the value of χ^2 would be 6·64 or less; in only 1% of cases would the value of χ^2 be as great as, or greater than 6·64, just due to chance. Since the value of χ^2 obtained (13·10) is greater than this, it is concluded that the observed and expected frequencies are significantly different. The null hypothesis that there is no difference between the success rates of the two techniques is rejected at the 1% level of significance. The success rate of the multiple-pressure method is significantly greater than the scratch method. In fact, in this particular example in only about 0·1% of cases would the value of χ^2 be as great as 13·10 just due to chance. This is the meaning of the term $P < 0.001$ below the table.

EXAMPLE 4.9

Learning test score related to peripheral arteriosclerosis

PALT Score	Vessel wall	
	Thick	Not thick
Less than 10	9	28
10–29	16	62
30 and over	16	17

$$\chi^2 = 9.43; P = 0.01$$

Reprinted from the *British Journal of Preventive and Social Medicine.* Parsons P. L. (1965), **19**, 43. Mental health of Swansea's old folk. (By permission of the Author, Editor, and Publishers.)

Another χ^2 test is shown in Example 4.9 in which the object is to determine whether or not the PALT (Paired Associates Learning Test) test score differs significantly between the two groups with regard to the degree of peripheral arteriosclerosis.

The null hypothesis asserts that any difference in the distribution of scores between the two groups arises by chance; the two groups have been drawn from identical populations with respect to the distribution of PALT scores. If the null hypothesis is true, the distribution of scores for the two groups should be similar. On this assumption the expected frequencies for each cell of the table are calculated and compared with the observed frequencies. From this comparison a value for χ^2 of 9·43 is obtained.

The table of the χ^2 distribution is then consulted. The number of degrees of freedom is two ($n = 2$). This may be verified by observing that given the marginal totals the maximum number of cells which can be filled independently is two. With $n = 2$, the value of χ^2 at the 1% level of significance is 9·21. This is interpreted to mean that, if the hypothesis were true, in only about 1 case in 100 would we expect to obtain a value of χ^2 as great as or greater than 9·21 just due to chance. The value of χ^2 obtained (9·43) is greater than this and is therefore significant at the 1% level; the null hypothesis is rejected. This is taken to mean that there is a significant difference in the distribution of scores between the two groups.

The χ^2 test is extensively used in medical research and is probably the most commonly used test of significance. Like the other tests referred to, the χ^2 test is based on the notion that if repeated samples are drawn from a population, the sample statistics will be distributed in a certain way around the population parameter. If the distribution of sample values is markedly different from the known or expected population distribution, it may be inferred that the sample differs significantly from the population, and could not have been drawn from that population. Or if two sample distributions are markedly different, it may be inferred that they could not have been drawn from the same population or from identical populations.

In this chapter some of the most important applications of statistical inference have been discussed. Many of the tests of significance referred to in articles in medical journals are covered by the examples given here, or by simple variations of these examples. In a later chapter some other types of tests of significance will be discussed involving other sampling distributions. At this stage, however, the reader should have a good grasp of the general principles and methods of application of tests of significance. It is then advisable before continuing further to read Chapters 3 and 4 again.

5

5.1 Regression lines and equations

In medical research it is often necessary to examine the relationship between a number of different variables—to determine whether a relationship exists and if so how close that relationship might be. For example, when a patient is admitted to hospital, particulars such as the patient's age, sex, occupation, weight, smoking experience and many other details which depend upon the form of illness of the patient are collected. These data may then be analysed in a number of ways, some of which have been described in previous chapters. A frequent aim of analysis, however, is to determine whether or not there is an association between the variables of interest. For instance, for a group of patients an association would be expected between height and weight. We would expect that, *on average*, taller patients would weigh more. Similarly, one might expect an association between coronary heart disease mortality and increasing age. If there appeared also to be a close association between coronary heart disease and cigarette smoking, this would be more interesting since it might provide some evidence of a *causal* link between the two.

Consider now the scatter diagram in Example 5.1. The construction of scatter diagrams was discussed in the first chapter and the reader should refer back to examples in that chapter. Example 5.1 shows the result of an experiment in which 100 readings were taken on an A.O. Haemoglobin meter and on an E.E.L. Colorimeter, and the results compared. Both instruments give very similar readings for each blood sample tested, and this is seen on the scatter diagram. The points on the scatter diagram show a clear trend, upwards and to the right; there is said to be a

EXAMPLE 5.1

Mean haemoglobin levels (as g Hb/100 ml blood) based on duplicate estimations made on an A.O. Haemoglobin meter and an E.E.L. Colorimeter.

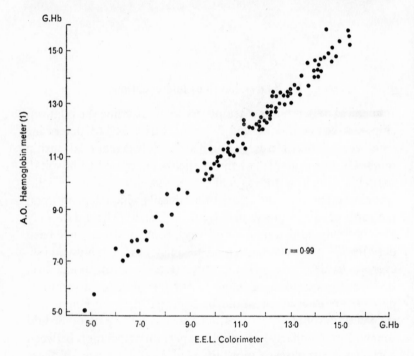

Reprinted from the *British Medical Journal*. Elwood P. C., and Jacobs A. (1966), **1**, 20. Haemoglobin estimation: A comparison of different techniques. (By permission of the Authors, Editor, and Publishers.)

direct or *positive* relationship between the two sets of readings. High (low) values of one variable are associated with high (low) values of the other.

A number of interesting questions now arise. First, is it possible to describe the numerical association between the two variables in some compact way? For example, suppose the two instruments always gave the same reading for any blood sample. Then denoting the E.E.L. Colorimeter reading by x, and the A.O. Haemoglobin meter reading by y, we could write the relationship as

$y = x$. Alternatively, if the A.O. Haemoglobin meter reading was always 90% of the E.E.L. Colorimeter reading, we could write the relationship as $y = 0.9x$. Given any value for an E.E.L. Colorimeter reading, we could be certain that the A.O. Haemoglobin meter reading would be 90% of that value. In this way, the relationship between the two variables is described by means of an equation.

Let us now return to Example 5.1. It is evident that although the association between the two variables is close, it is not as precise as that suggested by the formal mathematical equations above. Graphically, an equation of the form $y = x$, or $y = 0.9x$, can be represented by a straight line, and if the relationship between y and x were exact all the points on the scatter diagram would lie on this line. An example of this type of relationship is shown in Fig. 5.1.

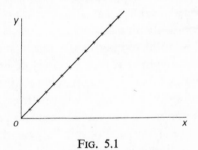

FIG. 5.1

All the points on the scatter diagram lie on a fixed line through the origin (O). The relationship between the two variables is 'exact' or 'perfect'.

More generally, the equation to a straight line may be expressed as $y = a + bx$, where 'a' is the intercept of the line on the y axis, and 'b' is the slope of the line. In the special case in which the line passes through the origin (O) of the two axes, as in Fig. 5.1, $a = 0$ and the line reduces to $y = bx$. The value of the coefficient b may take any positive value. In the equation $y = 0.9x$, for example, $b = 0.9$.

In Fig. 5.2, there is also a perfect association between x and y, but the trend is downwards to the right; there is said to be an *indirect* or *inverse* relationship between the two variables. In equation form such a relationship can also be written $y = a + bx$, although in this case the coefficient b would take a negative value, indicating that as one variable increased, the other decreased.

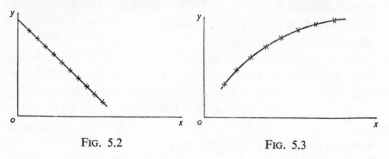

FIG. 5.2   FIG. 5.3

In Figs. 5.1 and 5.2, the points on the scatter diagram lie on a straight line, the relationship is said to be linear. In Fig. 5.3, the points also lie on a line, but the relationship is non-linear in form, and the equation to the line is more complex. However, there is still a 'perfect' relationship between x and y such that, given a value for x, the value for y can be precisely determined.

Finally, in Fig. 5.4 there is no apparent relationship between x and y. High values of x are associated with both high and low values of y. The points in the scatter show no particular 'trend' and, in the absence of any relationship between the two variables, the use of an equation is inappropriate.

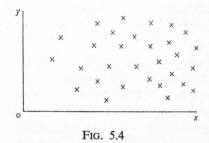

FIG. 5.4

When there is an obvious relationship between the two variables, as in Figs. 5.1 to 5.3, the relationship can be described by 'fitting a line' to the points on the scatter diagram. Algebraically, the line can be described by means of an equation. The line is called a *regression line* and the corresponding equation is called a *regression equation*. Figures 5.1 and 5.2 are examples of *linear* regression lines in which the relationship can be described by a straight line. Figure 5.3 is an example of a *curvi-linear* relationship where the regression line is non-linear; the corresponding regression equation would also be non-linear.

A regression line and its equation imply a numerical relationship between the two variables concerned. For example, the regression equation $y = 1 \cdot 5 + 2 \cdot 0x$ means that for any given value of x, an associated value for y can be calculated. It also suggests that an increase of 1 unit in x will be associated with an increase of 2 units in y. In Figs. 5.1 to 5.3 all the points in the scatter diagram lie on the regression line. This implies that the relationship between the two variables corresponds exactly to the relationship described by the regression equation.

Returning now to Example 5.1, it is clear that we cannot draw a linear regression line which will pass through *all* the points on the scatter. The relationship between actual or 'observed' pairs of readings of the Haemoglobin meter and the Colorimeter cannot conform exactly to the algebraic relationship described by a linear regression equation. However, the relationship seems to be approximately linear and, by using a ruler, a straight line can be superimposed on the scatter diagram. This is shown in Fig. 5.5.

The line passes through the middle of the scatter points. Few points lie on the line, but most lie close to the line, and the regression line might reasonably be claimed to represent approximately the relationship between the two variables.

The equation to a regression line fitted in this way can be written

$$y_c = a + bx$$

where y_c is the 'computed' or 'expected' value of y, given any value of x.

Thus, suppose the regression equation was

$$y_c = 0 \cdot 5 + 1 \cdot 1x$$

If $x = 10$, substitution in the regression equation tells us that the 'expected' value of y (y_c) would be 11·5 ($0·5 + 1·1 \times 10 = 11·5$). In practice, however, the observed or actual value of y corresponding to a value of $x = 10$ might be greater or less than this. This arises because the observed relationship between the two variables does not correspond exactly to the regression equation.

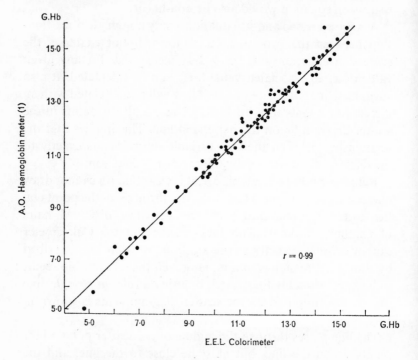

FIG. 5.5. Mean haemoglobin levels (as g Hg/100 ml blood) based on duplicate estimations made on an A.O. Haemoglobin meter and an E.E.L. Colorimeter.

To summarize, if the points on a scatter diagram suggest some association or relationship between two variables, it is possible to describe this relationship by means of a regression line and regression equation. The line and equation specify a numerical relationship between the two variables; given the value of one variable the value of the other can be estimated. However, except in rare cases, the observed relationship between the two variables will not correspond exactly to that expressed in the equation.

For the moment discussion will be confined to relationships between two variables, and to relationships which are linear in form. This involves what are called bi-variate linear regression lines.

5.2 Fitting regression lines

The methods used to fit regression lines will now be briefly discussed. Two examples of bi-variate linear regression lines are shown in Examples 5.2a and b.

EXAMPLE 5.2a

Relationship between mean birth weight and maternal height. Only means based on at least 100 observations have been entered on the diagram. The calculation of the regression line was based on all observations.

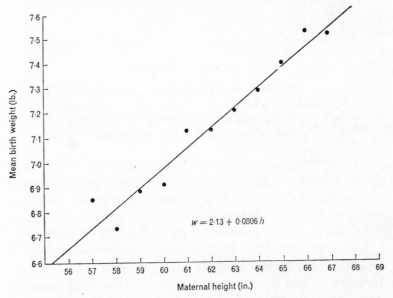

$$w = 2 \cdot 13 + 0 \cdot 0806 \, h$$

Reprinted from the *British Journal of Preventive and Social Medicine*. Barron S. L., and Vessey M. P. (1966), **20**, 127. Birth weight of infants born to immigrant women. By permission of the Authors, Editor, and Publishers.)

EXAMPLE 5.2b

Urinary oestriol excretion at 34th week of pregnancy in relation to gestation at onset of labour.

Coefficient of correlation, r, is negative.

Equation of regression: $y = 42\cdot7913 - 0\cdot1208x$.

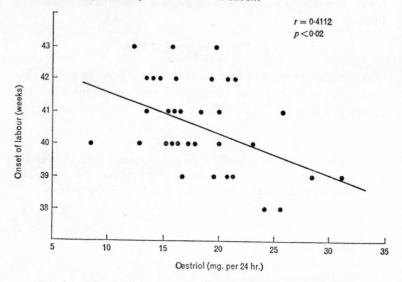

Reprinted from the *Lancet*. Turnbull A. C., Anderson A. B. M., and Wilson G. R. (1967), **2**, 627. Maternal urinary oestrogen excretion as evidence of a foetal role in determining gestation at labour. (By permission of the Authors, Editor, and Publishers.)

In Example 5.2a, there is obviously a direct relationship between maternal height (h) and mean birth-weight (w). In Example 5.2b there is an inverse relationship between oestriol and onset of labour. In both examples a regression line has been fitted to describe the relationship between the two variables.

Two questions now arise. Firstly, how is the regression line fitted? Secondly, how is the equation to the regression line obtained? These two questions will not be discussed in detail here, but the general principles involved in fitting regression lines and obtaining equations to the lines will be explained.

In the previous section it was suggested that a regression line could be fitted by hand, by drawing a line through the middle of the points on the scatter. Obviously this is a rather haphazard way of fitting the line and a more systematic procedure is required. A number of different methods can be used. For example, the line could be fitted by joining together the extreme points on the scatter. The best known method, however, is the method of 'least squares'.

Let us assume that the scatter of points is such that a straight line would be appropriate to describe the relationship. Among the infinite number of straight lines which could be drawn it is desirable to select that line to which the points on the scatter diagram are, in some sense, closest. That is, the line should be drawn in such a way as to minimize the distance between the scatter points and the line. In Fig. 5.6, the line has been fitted to

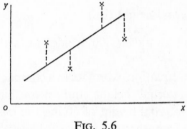

FIG. 5.6

minimize the sum of vertical distances between the four plot points and the line. Actually, since some of these distances will be positive (points above the line) and some will be negative (points below the line) the line is fitted to minimize the sum of the squares of the vertical distances between the plot points and the line.* This is why it is called the method of least squares.

When the line is fitted in this way, the overall difference between the plot points and the line is minimized. This is the line of 'best fit'. The actual methods by which the line is fitted need not be discussed here.

The regression lines in Examples 5.2a and b have been fitted by

---

* Since positive and negative distances would tend to cancel out, a regression line which was a 'poor fit' could still minimize the algebraic sum of the vertical distances between the plot points and the line. This is avoided by minimizing the *squares* of the distances, since all values are then positive.

the method of least squares. In Fig. 5.2a the plot points lie fairly close to the line. In Fig. 5.2b the points are dispersed more widely about the line. In both cases the sum of squares of vertical distances between the plot points and the line have been minimized. Given certain assumptions which will not be elaborated here, any point on the line represents the average value of one variable associated with a given value of the other.

Any straight line can be represented by a simple equation, and conversely. In Example 5.2a the equation corresponding to the regression line is written

$$w = 2 \cdot 13 + 0 \cdot 0806h$$

where w = mean birth-weight (lb)

h = maternal height (in.)

The coefficients $2 \cdot 13$ and $0 \cdot 0806$ are determined by the method of least squares.

This regression equation expresses in a compact way a relationship between maternal height and mean birth-weight. For example, for a maternal height of 60 in., the mean birth-weight can be estimated from the equation as follows:

$$w = 2 \cdot 13 + 0 \cdot 0806 \times 60$$
$$= 6 \cdot 966 \text{ lb}$$

On the regression line this is the point with co-ordinates 60 and $6 \cdot 966$. This can be interpreted to mean that, on average, we should expect a mother of height 60 in. to bear a baby of $6 \cdot 966$ lb. In practice the mean birth-weight may be more or less than this, but $6 \cdot 966$ is the *average* weight associated with a maternal height of 60 in.

The regression equation also implies that the average birth-weight will increase by $0 \cdot 0806$ lb with every increase of 1 in. in height. The coefficient $0 \cdot 0806$ in the equation is called the *regression coefficient*; it measures the change in w per unit change in h. It is equivalent to the slope of the regression line in Example 5.2a.

One further point may be noted. If a value of 0 is substituted for h, the value of w can be calculated as follows:

$$w = 2\cdot13 + 0\cdot0806 \times 0$$
$$= 2\cdot13 \text{ lb}$$

This suggests that a maternal height of zero is associated with a mean birth-weight of 2·13 lb. This is an absurd result. The regression equation is derived from observed values of the two variables, and it is only appropriate to describe the relationship between the two variables over a certain range of values. In Example 5.2a the regression equation can be regarded as relevant over the range 55–69 in. approximately.

The reader should now be able to interpret the regression equation of Example 5.2b which is written as follows:

$$y = 42\cdot7913 - 0\cdot1208x$$

where y = onset of labour (weeks), and

      x = oestriol excretion (mg/24 hr)

Here the regression coefficient is $-0\cdot1208$, which means that for every increase of 1 unit in x, the values of y decrease by 0·1208 units. This is to be expected as there is an inverse relationship between the two variables.

It is appropriate at this point to refer briefly to the question of causality or dependence between the variables in a regression equation. A regression equation expresses a numerical association between a pair of variables, but it does not imply any causal link between the two or prove that one variable is dependent upon another. It is, however, used to support an hypothesis of dependence of one variable upon another.

In Example 5.2a the hypothesis is that mean birth-weight is dependent, wholly or partly, on maternal height. Mean birth-weight is regarded as the *dependent* variable and maternal height as the *independent* variable. In the regression equation, the dependent variable is written on the left-hand side of the equation, and the independent variable on the right-hand side. Mathematically, however, the regression equation is unaltered by writing it as follows:

$$w - 0.0806h = 2.13$$

or

$$h = -26.43 + 12.41w$$

Writing the equation as

$$w = 2.13 + 0.0806h$$

indicates that w is to be regarded as dependent on h, and that the coefficients have been estimated in a certain way. The question of dependence or causality will be referred to again in a later section of this chapter.

So far the examples illustrated have related to linear relationships between variables. Non-linear relationships can be described in a similar way by fitting non-linear regression lines to the plot points and deriving equations for the lines. Non-linear regression equations will not be discussed here since they are often rather complex in form, but in principle they correspond to equations of linear type.

Example 5.3 illustrates how a non-linear relationship can be converted to linear form. The purpose of the enquiry is to investigate the relationship between cold weather and ischaemic heart disease mortality. Mean monthly temperature, over a period of years, is recorded on the abscissa. The ordinate records values of the 'monthly mortality index' which is defined as the ratio of the mean daily deaths for a particular month to the mean daily deaths for the corresponding year. This index, however, is expressed logarithmically so that the ordinate records *proportionate* changes in the mortality index. (The interpretation of a logarithmic scale was discussed in Chapter 1.) The resulting scatter diagram shows the relationship between changes in mean monthly temperature and proportionate changes in mortality, and suggests a linear or near-linear inverse relationship. The use of logarithms to convert non-linear relationships to linear form is frequently used in regression analysis.

EXAMPLE 5.3

Relation between 'log monthly mortality index' for ASHD (males) and mean temperature (°F) for each month of the period 1958–62.

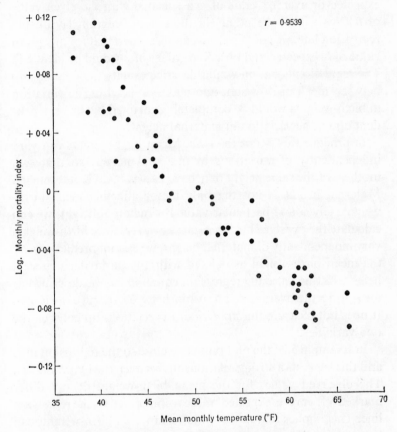

Reprinted from the *British Journal of Preventive and Social Medicine*. Rose G. (1966), **20**, 97. Cold weather and ischaemic heart disease. (By permission of the Author, Editor, and Publishers.)

5.3 Measures of correlation

The regression equation has been described as a measure of the *average* relationship between two variables. This is a rather vague description and must now be elaborated.

Consider the regression equation of Example 5.2a. For a given value of h (maternal height) a corresponding value of w can be calculated, which can be written $\hat{w}$. $\hat{w}$ can be interpreted as the expected or average value of w associated with the given value of h. Now, if all the points in the scatter diagram lay on the regression line, we could be reasonably certain that for any given value of h, expected and observed values of w would be identical. The regression equation would describe exactly the relationship between mean birth-weight and maternal height. The variation in birth-weights would be completely explained by, or be dependent upon, the variation in maternal height.

In practice this is not the case. Mean birth-weights can vary independently of variations in maternal height, so that two mothers of the same height may have babies of different weights. Maternal height is not the only factor affecting mean birth-weight. Given any particular value for maternal height, we can calculate the *expected* birth-weight; however, since birth-weights vary independently of maternal height, we cannot predict *exactly* the mean birth-weight associated with any particular maternal height. In this sense the regression equation can be described as measuring the average relationship between the two variables. It does not measure the *strength* of the relationship between the two variables.

In Example 5.2a the plot points lie close to the regression line, and this suggests a strong relationship between the two variables. The observed values for the mean birth-weight do not differ markedly from the 'expected' values represented by the regression line. This implies that most of the variation in birth-weights can be 'explained' by the variation in maternal height. Given a value for maternal height, we could estimate the expected birth-weight and be fairly sure that the actual birth-weight would be quite close to this in value.

In Example 5.2b, on the other hand, there is considerable variation in the dispersion of plot points around the regression line. This suggests a fairly weak relationship between the two variables. Given a value for oestriol at the 34th week of pregnancy, we could estimate the onset of labour, but the actual onset of labour could vary quite appreciably from this. A considerable amount of the variation in y is 'unexplained' by the variation in x. Although on average, y decreases with increasing x, there are obviously other factors which influence onset of labour.

A measure of the strength of the relationship between two variables is provided by the coefficient of correlation, denoted by 'r'. If the relationship between the two variables is of linear form, r is a measure of the *coefficient of linear correlation*.

Values of r vary between $+1$ and -1, the sign of r depending on whether or not there is a direct relationship between the two variables as in Example 5.2a, or an inverse relationship as in Example 5.2b. If the relationship between the two variables is perfect, that is if all the points on the scatter diagram lie on the regression line, r will be equal to $+1$ or -1. A positive sign indicates a direct relationship, a negative sign indicates an inverse one. If there is no relationship between the two variables, as in Fig. 5.4, r will be 0 or very nearly 0. The greater the numerical value of r, the stronger the relationship between the two variables.

The calculation of the coefficient of linear correlation will not be explained in detail here, but the general line of reasoning underlying the measure will be described using Example 5.2a as a reference. The variation in mean birth-weight is due partly to variations in maternal height (the 'explained' variation) and partly to other factors which have not been considered or are unknown (the 'unexplained' variation). The larger the first component is, relative to the second, the stronger is the relationship between the two variables.

The coefficient of linear correlation is calculated by estimating the proportion of the total variation in the dependent variable which is explained by the regression equation. If the total variation is written as 1, the proportion of the total variation which is explained by the regression line is written as r^2. If the relationship between the two variables is perfect all the variation in the dependent variable is explained by the regression line, and $r^2 = 1$, so that $r = 1$. Then r is written plus or minus according to whether the relationship is direct or inverse. The more closely the points in the scatter diagram are dispersed around the regression line, the higher will be the proportion of the variation explained by the regression line, and hence the greater the value of r^2 and r.

EXAMPLE 5.4

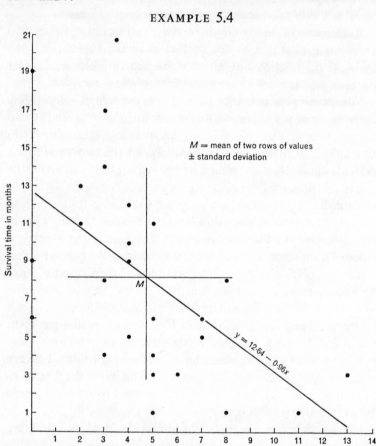

Reprinted from the *British Medical Journal*. Halikowski B., Armata J., and Garwicz S. (1966), **1**, 519. Low-protein purine-free diet in treatment of acute leukaemia in children: Preliminary communication. (By permission of the Authors, Editor, and Publishers.)

Consider now Example 5.4. The relationship between size of liver and survival time in months is plotted for 26 cases of acute leukaemia in children. A linear regression line is fitted to this data, giving the regression equation

$$y = 12 \cdot 64 - 0 \cdot 96x$$

where y = survival time in months and x = size of liver (cm).

There is an inverse relationship between the two variables. The regression coefficient is $-0 \cdot 96$. This means that, on average, an increase of 1 cm in liver size reduces the survival time, the dependent variable, by almost 1 month.

How strong is the relationship between survival and liver size? It will be observed that the plot points vary quite widely around the regression line. The five cases with liver size of 4 cm for instance, vary between 5 months and 21 months in survival time, as compared with an expected survival of $8 \cdot 8$ months from the regression equation. There is therefore quite a marked degree of variation in survival time which is not explained by the regression line.

The coefficient of linear correlation between survival time and size of liver is calculated and found to be $-0 \cdot 54$. The negative value indicates an inverse relationship. Since $r = -0 \cdot 54$, $r^2 = 0 \cdot 2916$. This may be interpreted to mean that about 29% of the variation in survival time is due to variation in liver size. The other 71% of the variation is 'unexplained'.

Returning to an earlier example, it will be noticed that in the scatter diagram of Example 5.2b a value for $r = -0 \cdot 4112$ is included. From this $r^2 = 0 \cdot 1691$ which means that about 17% of the variation in onset of labour is 'explained' by the variation in oestriol excretion. There is a fairly weak relationship between the two variables, as the scatter diagram suggests.

The coefficient of correlation is an important measure. The strength of the relationship between two variables is often of greater interest than the form of the relationship between them. In most cases involving the use of regression analysis, it is advisable to include the value of the correlation coefficient. In Example 5.1, at the beginning of the chapter, the regression line has been omitted altogether, but the coefficient of linear correlation is included. Here $r = +0 \cdot 99$, indicating a very strong relationship between the two sets of readings ($r^2 = 0.98$).

One further important point relating to the calculation of regression coefficients and correlation coefficients must now be explained. In the examples so far quoted, and in general, analysis is based on a *sample* of the pairs of variables of interest. Thus, Example 5.2a is a sample of maternity cases. Now, in the same way that the mean and standard deviation of a random sample are estimates of the mean and standard deviation of the population from which it was drawn, so the regression coefficient and correlation coefficient of a sample of pairs of two variables are estimates of the regression coefficient and correlation coefficient for the population of pairs of these values. Let the regression coefficient for the sample be denoted by b, and the correlation coefficient by r; similarly denote the regression coefficient for the whole population by β (beta), and the correlation coefficient by ρ (rho). Then the sample statistics b and r are estimates of the unknown population parameters β and ρ.

It will be recalled that in Chapter 3 it was explained how 95% confidence limits for an estimate of the population mean could be obtained using the sample mean and standard error. Similarly, having calculated b and r from a sample, confidence limits for estimates of β and ρ can be obtained by calculating the standard errors of estimate for b and r.

An interesting possibility now arises. Suppose, for the whole population of pairs of values, $\beta = 0$ and $\rho = 0$. This would occur in cases where, as in Fig. 5.4, there is no relationship between the two variables.* The two variables are said to be independent of one another. An example would be pairs of values which arise in throwing two dice simultaneously. There is no relationship (or should not be!) between the number which turns up on one die and the number turning up on the other. A regression analysis between pairs of values should yield $\beta = 0$ and $\rho = 0$.

---

* β is a measure of the average change in one variable (y) per unit change in the other (x). If there is no relationship between x and y, an increase of one unit in x is equally likely to be associated with a decrease or increase in y. Hence, the *average* change in y per unit change in x will be 0. Similarly, if no relationship can be postulated between x and y, $\rho = 0$.

However, if a sample of pairs of values is analysed, it is quite possible that, just by chance, non-zero values will be obtained for b and r. In the same way that the mean $(\bar{X})$ of a single sample is unlikely to be exactly equal to the population mean (μ), the values of the regression coefficient b and the correlation coefficient r derived from a sample are unlikely to be exactly equal to the population values β and ρ. Hence, it is likely that even if β and $\rho = 0$, b and r will be non-zero. This means that the results of the regression analysis may suggest a relationship between two variables which is quite spurious.

To guard against this possibility, some method must be devised to test the significance of the values of b and r obtained. Such a method is available, and is very similar to the tests of significance already described. The object of the test is to determine whether or not the value of r (and b) obtained is significantly different from zero. As in previous tests of significance involving sample statistics and population parameters the null hypothesis is used; this states that the value of r obtained differs from zero only by chance. The hypothesis is tested by calculating the probability of obtaining a value of r as great as the one obtained, just by chance. If this probability is very small, say less than 0·05, the null hypothesis is rejected. The value of r obtained is said to be significantly different from zero and an association between the two variables is accepted.

The greater the value of r, the more likely it is that r, and hence ρ, differ significantly from zero. Unless the sample is very small, it is unlikely that a value of r as high as 0·9 could have arisen by chance. On the other hand, a value of r of 0·1 could quite easily arise by chance which is consistent with a value of $\rho = 0$. It is therefore important when calculating a correlation coefficient, and a regression coefficient, to test the significance of the values obtained. If these values are not significantly different from zero, no valid conclusions can be drawn from the results of the analysis.

Example 5.5 shows the results of an analysis of the relation between oxygen consumption (y) and temperature gradient between foot skin and incubator roof (x). A linear regression of

y (the dependent variable) on x yields the regression equation

$$y = 3.97 + 0.73x$$

The regression coefficient $b = 0.73$; an increase of 1 unit in temperature gradient is associated with an average increase of 0.73 in oxygen consumption.

The strength of the relationship between the two variables is given by $r = 0.66$, $r^2 = 0.4356$, so that approximately 44% of the variation in oxygen consumption is 'explained' by the variation in temperature gradient.

The null hypothesis is now applied to test the significance of the coefficient of correlation. The result of the test shows that if the null hypothesis were true (that $\rho = 0$), a value of r as great as, or greater than 0.66 would arise in less than 1 case in 100, just by chance. This is the meaning of the expression $t_r < 0.01$ in the example. Since this probability is very small, the null hypothesis is rejected; the value of r obtained, and hence ρ, is significantly different from zero. Referring back to Example 5.4, the value of the correlation coefficient is -0.54 and this is also shown to be significantly different from zero. If the null hypothesis were true, that $\rho = 0$, a value of r as great as, or greater than, 0.54 would arise by chance in only one or two cases in 100; the probability of obtaining such a value of 0.54 by chance would be between 0.01 and 0.02. The value of r obtained is significantly different from 0 at the 5%, and 2%, levels of significance, though it is not significantly different from 0 at the 1% level.

5.4 Association and dependence

In an earlier section it was explained that in fitting regression lines one variable is regarded as dependent on another. Usually the direction of the dependence is obvious. Thus, in Example 5.2a it is clear that mean birth-weight is dependent on maternal height, and it would be absurd to regard maternal height as dependent on mean birth-weight.

In other cases, however, the form of relationship may be less obvious; indeed the two variables may be independent but

EXAMPLE 5.5

Relation between oxygen consumption (S.T.P.D.) and temperature gradient between foot skin and incubator roof.

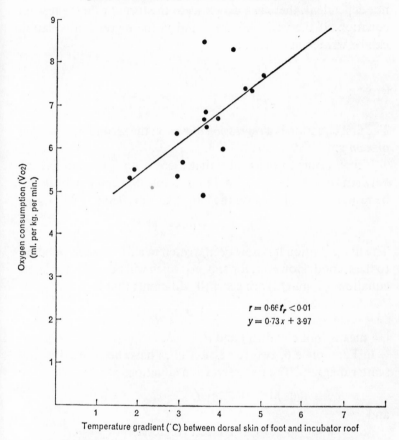

$r = 0.66$ $t_r < 0.01$
$y = 0.73x + 3.97$

Oxygen consumption ($\dot{V}o_2$) (ml. per kg. per min.)

Temperature gradient (°C) between dorsal skin of foot and incubator roof

Reprinted from the *Lancet*. Levison H., Linsao L., and Swyer P. R. (1966), **2**, 1346. A comparison of infra-red and convective heating for newborn infants. (By permission of the Authors, Editor, and Publishers.)

apparently correlated through their mutual dependence on some other factor. In Example 5.1, the A.O. Haemoglobin meter and the E.E.L. Colorimeter readings are not dependent upon one another in any sense; they are closely associated as both purport to measure haemoglobin levels for the same group of blood samples.

In cases of this kind, where the variables are associated but not dependent, there is a choice as to the form of the regression equation. If the variables are x and y, the regression equation can be written as follows:

$$(1) \quad y = a + bx$$

or as

$$(2) \quad x = c + dy$$

The first equation is a *regression of y on x*; the second a *regression of x on y*.

It may occur to the reader that there is no formal difference between these two equations. For example, the first equation can be re-written to place x on the left-hand side. Thus,

$$(3) \quad x = -a/b + (1/b)y$$

The first equation has now been written in a form corresponding to the second. However, for reasons which will be explained later, equations (2) and (3) are generally different; that is

$$c \neq -a/b$$

($\neq$ means 'not equal to') and $d \neq 1/b$.

In Example 5.6, two regression lines have been fitted to the scatter diagram. The two regression equations are

$$x = 0.0874 + 0.8724y \text{ (regression of } x \text{ on } y)$$

and

$$y = -0.0613 + 1.1135x \text{ (regression of } y \text{ on } x)$$

The two regression lines, though close together, are not identical. Since both equations measure the relationship between x and y, it may be thought odd that the two regression lines are different. However, this is because the two lines are fitted by different methods. The first is fitted by minimizing the sum of squares of the *horizontal* distances between the plot points and the regression line. The second line is fitted by minimizing the sum of squares of the *vertical* distances between the plot points

EXAMPLE 5.6

Regression lines (x on y and y on x) for the ratio of octanoic-acid concentration (0–60 μg per ml) to 20 μg nonanoic acid per ml and the ratio of the peak heights on the gas/liquid chromatogram. $x = 0.0874 + 0.8724y$; $y = -0.0613 + 1.1135x$.

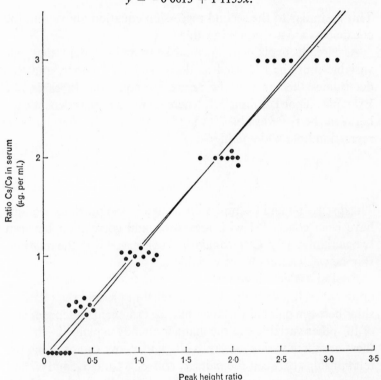

Reprinted from the *Lancet*. Linscheer W. G., Slone D., and Chalmers T. C. (1967), **1**, 593, Effects of octanoic acid on serum-levels of free fatty acids, insulin, and glucose in patients with cirrhosis and in healthy volunteers. (By permission of the Authors, Editor, and Publishers.)

and the regression line (see Example 5.6). Unless the relationship between the two variables is perfect, the two regression lines fitted by these two methods will be different. The stronger the relationship between the two variables, the closer will be the two regression lines.

As an illustration, the first regression equation above can be re-written to put y on the left-hand side of the equation. This gives

$$y = -0\cdot1002 + 1\cdot1463x$$

This is similar to the second regression equation above, but the coefficients are not equal in value.

As already explained, in most cases it is evident that one variable must be regarded as dependent on another, and this determines the form of the regression equation. In cases like Example 5.6, or Example 5.1, where there is no clear dependence between the two variables it may be desirable to compute both regression lines and equations.

5.5 Multiple regression

The discussion and examples illustrated in the previous sections have been concerned with regression and correlation between two variables only. Often analysis is concerned with the relationship between a number of variables.

Analysis which involves more than two variables may be approached in two ways. Using the first approach, the relationships between pairs of variables may be examined, independently of the other variables, in the manner already explained. Thus, if there are three variables, say x_1, x_2, and x_3, we can examine the relationships between the pairs x_1 and x_2, x_2 and x_3, and x_1 and x_3, in each case ignoring the third variable. An example of this kind of analysis is shown in Example 5.7.

There are five variables in this example, and the figures in the table refer to the values of the correlation coefficients between any pair of variables. Thus, in the first line the coefficient of correlation between systolic and diastolic blood pressure is $0\cdot6337$; the coefficient of correlation between systolic blood pressure and age is $0\cdot2405$, and so on. In the second line the coefficient of correlation between diastolic and systolic blood pressure is omitted since it already appears in the first line. The coefficient of correlation between diastolic blood pressure and age is 0·0290, and so on. The figures '1' shown in the diagonal of the table may be ignored.

Each correlation coefficient is calculated between two variables, quite independently of the other three variables. The table therefore consists of a number of separate bi-variate correlation coefficients calculated by the methods described in Section 5.3, and interpreted in the same way. Each correlation coefficient has been tested for significance and those correlation coefficients which are significantly different from 0, at the 5% level of significance, are marked with an asterisk.

EXAMPLE 5.7

Zero order correlation coefficients between systolic pressure, diastolic pressure, age, body weight, and arm circumference

Variable	Variable				
	Systolic	Diastolic	Age	Weight	Arm
Systolic	1	0·6337*	0·2405*	−0·0715	−0·0918
Diastolic		1	0·0290	0·0187	0·0316
Age			1	−0·1311	−0·2178*
Weight				1	0·6058*
Arm					1

Reprinted from the *British Journal of Preventive and Social Medicine*. Khosla T., and Lowe C. R. (1965), **19**, 159. Arterial pressure and arm circumference. (Table abbreviated.) (By permission of the Authors, Editor, and Publishers.)

A table of this kind, sometimes referred to as a matrix of bi-variate correlation coefficients, is a useful method of summarizing the independent relationships between a number of variables, and of showing which relationships are significant. In Example 5.7, there are four significant (*) relationships. The remaining correlations can be ignored.

The second approach to be described is quite different, involving the simultaneous analysis of a number of variables. This is called *multiple regression analysis*, as distinct from simple bi-variate analysis which deals only with two variables.

As an example, an individual's weight depends on a number of factors including his height and his average carbohydrate intake. Suppose we wished to examine the combined effect of height and average carbohydrate intake on weight. Assuming a linear relationship, this could be expressed as:

$$y = a + b_1 x_1 + b_2 x_2$$

where y = weight

x_1 = height

x_2 = average carbohydrate intake.

In this multiple regression equation, y is the dependent variable and x_1 and x_2 are independent or explanatory variables. The coefficients b_1 and b_2 are called *partial regression coefficients*; b_1 is a measure of the average change in y per unit change in x_1, with x_2 constant, and b_2 is a measure of the average change in y per unit change in x_2, with x_1 constant.

A multiple regression equation of this form can be fitted to observed data by methods similar to those used for simple bi-variate regression. If the reader can envisage a three-dimensional scatter diagram, the regression plane is fitted to the data as before as the plane of 'best fit'. The partial regression coefficients are calculated, as well as the constant a, and the equation describes the average relationship between the dependent variable and the independent variables. In principle, there is no limit to the number of independent variables which may be included.

Example 5.8 shows the results of a number of multiple regression analyses. The left-hand side of the table shows the relationship between systolic blood pressure, the dependent variable, and age and body weight, the explanatory variables. Data were collected by five different observers so that five separate regressions could be calculated. For Observer A, the multiple regression equation for systolic blood pressure on age and weight could be written

$$y = a + 3 \cdot 57x_1 - 0 \cdot 03x_2$$

where y = systolic blood pressure (mm)

       x_1 = age in units of 5 years

       x_2 = body weight (lb)

The equation suggests that systolic blood pressure will increase, on average, by 3·57 mm every 5 years, and will decrease by about 0·03 mm with every lb increase in body weight. The value of a, in this example, is unimportant.

EXAMPLE 5.8

Mean and partial regression coefficients for systolic and diastolic pressures in respect of age and weight

Observer	Mean (mm)	Systolic *(dep)* b_1 mm per 5 years	b_2 *(indep)* mm per lb	Mean (mm)	Diastolic b_1 mm per 5 years	b_2 mm per lb
A	127·3	3·57*	−0·03	83·8	0·27	0·01
B	137·9	4·67*	0·16*	81·2	0·91	0·12*
C	140·4	4·61*	0·11	83·9	1·65	0·08*
D	141·7	8·16*	0·08	81·8	2·57*	0·10*
E	143·5	5·05*	0·39*	81·8	1·30	0·23*

Reprinted from the *British Journal of Preventive and Social Medicine*. Khosla T., and Lowe C. R. (1965), **19**, 159. Arterial pressure and arm circumference. (By permission of the Authors, Editor, and Publishers.)

However, when the partial regression coefficients are tested for significance, it is found that only the partial regression coefficient for age (3·57) is significantly different from zero which implies that body weight has no significant effect on systolic blood pressure.

When the results for the other observers are considered, age is seen to be significant in each case, although there is a marked variation in the values of the partial regression coefficients presumably reflecting observer bias. In the case of body weight, the partial regression coefficients also varied considerably and in two cases (Observers B and E) the value of the partial regression coefficient was found to be significantly different from zero.

The results for the regression of diastolic blood pressure on age and body weight may be similarly interpreted by the reader. It will be noted that age appears to be less important with respect to diastolic blood pressure; in only one case is the partial regression coefficient significantly different from zero. On the other hand body weight appears to be more important. Values marked with an asterisk are significantly different from zero at the 5% level.

The strength of the relationship between the dependent variable and the explanatory variables may also be estimated by calculating the *coefficient of multiple correlation*. As before, r^2 measures the proportion of the total variation in the dependent variable which can be 'explained' by variations in the explanatory variables. The 'unexplained' variation may be due, of course, to other variables which have not been included in the regression equation. If these variables can be identified then a new multiple regression equation can be calculated with these additional variables included. The value of r, and r^2, will be increased since the proportion of 'explained' variation in the dependent variable will be higher. Moreover, by calculating what are called *partial correlation coefficients*, the strength of the relationship between the dependent variable and any one of the independent variables may be calculated, assuming the other independent variables are held constant. These partial correlation coefficients differ from the simple bi-variate (or zero-order) correlation coefficients described on pp. 114–15. In the former, the simultaneous influence of other independent variables is taken into account. In the latter, the correlation between two variables is calculated without any explicit attempt to remove the possible influence of other variables.

In multiple regression analysis interest lies in the variation in one variable called the dependent variable. Multivariate analysis is designed to handle cases of simultaneous variation in two or more dependent variables. Multivariate problems are common in medical research and in recent years there has been a substantial development in statistical techniques and applications of multivariate analysis. An example is *discriminant analysis*. Suppose two populations are defined by a set of characteristics such as height, weight, serum cholesterol level, etc. Suppose also that for each characteristic the two distributions overlap, so that for example the distribution of heights in population A overlaps with the distribution of heights in population B. Thus, although the mean height of individuals in population A may be less than the mean height of individuals in population B, one individual picked at random from population A may be taller than an individual picked at random from population B. Consequently, if we encountered an individual and did not know which population that individual belonged to, we could not definitely assign him to a particular population, unless for any one of the variables concerned the distributions were known not to overlap.

The purpose of discriminant analysis is to enable us to assign individual units to one or other of the populations with, in some defined sense, the greatest probability of being correct (or smallest risk of error). The techniques of analysis, which will not be explained here, involve the specification of a discriminant function in which the relevant variables are assigned a weight, or coefficient. If the discriminant function is linear in form it will 'look like' a multiple regression equation. For a particular individual or case, values of the variables (height, weight, etc.) are substituted in the discriminant equation and a value for the function calculated. On the basis of this value the individual is assigned to a particular population.

As an indication of the possible application of discriminant analysis, suppose it is desired to allocate individuals to a 'high risk' or 'low risk' category for a particular disease, the allocation being made on the basis of certain diagnostic variables, e.g. blood pressure, age. Coefficients of the discriminant function are estimated using sample observations of those who have, and those who have not, contracted the disease in some past period. Individuals can then be assigned to one or other category using the discriminant function as the method of allocation. A good example of the use of discriminant analysis for this purpose is the study of risk factors in coronary heart disease in Framingham (Truett J., Cornfield J., and Kannel W., 1967, A multivariate analysis of the risk of coronary heart disease in Framingham, *J. chron. Dis.* **20**, 511).

5.6   Rank correlation

A rather different type of measure of correlation will now be described. Suppose ten children are subjected to a form of intelligence test by two independent assessors. Since it is not easy to determine intelligence by means of an objective numerical measure, it may be found more convenient to *rank* the children in an order corresponding to their alleged degree of intelligence, as in the following example.

EXAMPLE 5.9

Child	1	2	3	4	5	6	7	8	9	10
Investigator A	7	6	1	2	3	9	9	10	4	5
Investigator B	6	7	3	2	1	4	9	8	10	5

The ranking order, though similar, is different. It may be of interest to assess the degree of concordance, or correlation, between the ranking order of the two investigators.

If the ranking orders were exactly the same we should expect a coefficient of correlation of $+1$. On the other hand, if the ranking order of Investigator B were exactly the *reverse* of Investigator A we should expect the coefficient of correlation to be -1. If there is no relationship at all between the two rankings we should expect the coefficient of correlation to be 0, or almost 0.

A measure of correlation, called Spearman's *rank correlation coefficient*, has been devised for this purpose. The calculation of this rank correlation coefficient will not be explained here; it is based on the difference in ranking order. In the example quoted here, Spearman's rank correlation coefficient is $r = +0.54$, which can be shown to be significantly different from zero. There is a significant degree of correlation between the ranking orders of the two Investigators.

In cases where more than two ranking orders are to be compared, a similar measure called the coefficient of concordance may be calculated, and other measures based on ranking are available for more complex problems. Measures of rank correlation and other rank tests are examples of non-parametric or distribution-free tests, since they do not involve particular assumptions about the form of the parent populations from which the samples are drawn. The particular application of the χ^2 distribution discussed in Chapter 4 is also a non-parametric test, though other applications involving the χ^2 distribution are dependent upon assumed properties of the parent population, e.g. normality.

In this chapter it has been explained how the relationship between a number of variables may be described by means of a regression equation and how the strength of the relationship between the variables may be measured. In addition it has been shown how the significance of statistics such as the regression coefficient and the correlation coefficient may be tested. It is appropriate to complete this chapter with a word of caution concerning the interpretation of measures of regression and correlation. The establishment of a functional relationship, in the form of a regression equation, between one variable and another or others, does not establish a *causal* link between the variables concerned. It is possible to establish a positive relationship between the growth of private vehicle registrations in Ireland and the annual average number of telephone calls in Ireland; both may reflect a more affluent society but it is not suggested that there is a causal link between the two. Both may depend on a third factor, such as income, but be independent of one another. Many variables move in the same direction, or in opposite directions, over time without being in any way causally related. In practice, measures of regression and correlation are used to support hypotheses of causality, but they cannot of themselves provide *proof* of causal relationships.

6

6.1 Introduction

In previous chapters some of the important applications of statistical inference were discussed, and examples were given of their application to medical research problems. There are, of course, a considerable variety of such applications which are available to the statistician, based upon principles of statistical inference. The objective in this book has been to present and discuss general concepts and methods of reasoning which underlie statistical analysis; and while the reader may not be familiar with the precise statistical or mathematical techniques used in a particular problem, it is hoped that the logic of the procedure and the results may be generally understood.

In this chapter, a miscellany of topics will be discussed. In Sections 6.2 to 6.6 further extensions and applications of statistical inference and tests of significance are discussed. Some of these topics, such as sequential analysis and analysis of variance are quite complex and, at an introductory level discussion is necessarily brief and general. However, the reader should now be able to follow the basic methodology of these techniques.

6.2 One-tailed tests of significance

Consider the following hypothetical problem.

It is asserted that the cholesterol level of agricultural labourers is higher than that of the general male population. A stratified* random sample of 100 agricultural labourers results in a mean cholesterol level of 249·0. From other sources it is known that

---

* Stratified by age groups.

the mean cholesterol level for the general male population is 241·0, with a standard deviation of 45·0. Does this evidence support the assertion?

From the data above, the standard error can be shown to be $45/\sqrt{100} = 4\cdot5$. Hence, with $\mu = 241\cdot0$, the 95% confidence interval for $\bar{X}$ can be calculated as

$$\mu \pm 1\cdot96\sigma_{\bar{X}} = 241\cdot0 \pm 1\cdot96 \times 4\cdot5$$
$$= 241\cdot0 \pm 8\cdot82$$
$$= 232\cdot18 \text{ to } 249\cdot82.$$

The value of $\bar{X}$ obtained, which is 249·0, falls inside this 95% range, and we might therefore conclude that there is not a significant difference between $\bar{X}$ and μ—the cholesterol level of agricultural labourers is not significantly different from the cholesterol level for the whole male population.

However, in this particular problem it is asserted that, whatever the mean cholesterol level of agricultural labourers might be, it will certainly not be significantly *less* than the mean cholesterol level for the general male population. Hence, if the mean cholesterol level of the sample of 100 agricultural labourers had turned out to be 232·0, instead of 249·0, we should have attributed this to chance. We would not have concluded that the mean cholesterol level of agricultural labourers was significantly *less* than the mean cholesterol level for the general male population, even though the sample mean fell below the 95% confidence interval.

This type of problem involves the use of a *one-tailed test* as distinct from the *two-tailed test* described in Chapters 3 and 4. The basis of the two-tailed test is shown in Fig. 6.1a below. Using a 5% level of significance, the critical area is shown by the two shaded 'tails' of the distribution, each of which accounts for $2\frac{1}{2}\%$ of the area under the normal curve. l_1 and l_2 mark the limits of the 95% confidence interval. The null hypothesis is rejected if $\bar{X}$ falls above l_2 *or* below l_1. The hypothesis is accepted if $\bar{X}$ falls between l_1 and l_2—that is, within the 95% confidence interval.

Figure 6.1b, in contrast, illustrates the basis of a one-tailed

I

test. Using a 5% level of significance, the critical area is the shaded area at the upper tail of the distribution. The lower tail is not used, since it is asserted that *any value of $\bar{X}$ less than μ is not significantly different from μ.*

In this case, the critical limit l_2 is given by $\mu + 1\cdot64\sigma_{\bar{X}}$, which cuts off the upper 5% of the area under the curve, and not by $\mu + 1\cdot96\sigma_{\bar{X}}$, which cuts off the upper $2\frac{1}{2}\%$ of the area under the curve. If $\bar{X}$ falls above l_2 the null hypothesis is rejected. If $\bar{X}$ falls below l_2 the null hypothesis is accepted. There is no lower limit to the 95% confidence interval.

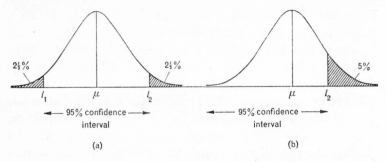

FIG. 6.1

Similarly, if a 1% level of significance is used, the critical upper limit is found as $\mu + 2\cdot33\sigma_{\bar{X}}$, and not as $\mu + 2\cdot58\sigma_{\bar{X}}$. If $\bar{X}$ falls above the critical upper limit determined from $\mu + 2\cdot33\sigma_{\bar{X}}$, the null hypothesis is rejected, while any value of $\bar{X}$ below the limit is consistent with the null hypothesis. The 99% confidence interval has a critical upper limit but no lower limit. The one-tailed test may also be applied if it is only values of $\bar{X}$ *below* a certain critical limit which are of interest. In this case the critical lower limit l_1, using a 5% level of significance is $\mu - 1\cdot64\sigma_{\bar{X}}$. If a 1% level of significance (99% confidence interval) is used, the critical lower limit is found as $\mu - 2\cdot33\sigma_{\bar{X}}$.

Returning now to the example above, it is clear that only values of $\bar{X}$ which are greater than μ are of interest. A one-tailed test is appropriate. Using a 5% level of significance, the critical upper limit for $\bar{X}$ is given by

$$\mu + 1\cdot64\sigma_{\bar{X}} = 241\cdot0 + 1\cdot64 \times 4\cdot5$$
$$= 241\cdot0 + 7\cdot38$$
$$= 248\cdot38.$$

Since the value of $\bar{X}$ obtained (249.0) falls above this critical value, we are justified in rejecting the null hypothesis at the 5% level of significance—we conclude that the cholesterol level of agricultural labourers is significantly higher than that of the general male population.

However, the reader may care to verify that the difference between $\bar{X}$ and μ in this problem is not significant at the 1% level, by calculating the critical upper limit $\mu + 2\cdot33\sigma_{\bar{X}}$, and noting that $\bar{X}$ falls within the corresponding 99% confidence interval. The difference between μ and $\bar{X}$ is significant at the 5% level ($P < 0\cdot05$) but not significant at the 1% level ($P > 0\cdot01$).

One-tailed tests are commonly used in scientific research problems where the result is expected in one direction only. An example would be a drug/placebo trial where one would normally expect the result to favour the active compound. Depending on the circumstances, however, a two-tailed test might still be preferred if the experimenter wants to retain the right to *reject* the active compound, rather than simply to say it is no better than the placebo.

6.3 Dichotomous populations

Populations may often be classified by whether or not the units in that population possess a certain attribute or characteristic. For example, a population may be divided into smokers and non-smokers, males or females, persons over 60 years of age and under 60 years of age, and so on. Such populations are called *dichotomous populations*, and involve the use of *proportions*. The application of the principles of statistical inference to proportions introduces a particular probability distribution called the *binomial distribution*.

In a dichotomous population, the population is divided into two categories. If the proportion falling into one category is written π (pi), then the proportion falling into the other category is $(1 - \pi)$. Thus, if 75% of the adult Irish male population are smokers, we could write $\pi = 0.75$, hence $(1 - \pi) = 0.25$. Moreover, the probability that an adult male selected at random from this population will be a smoker is 0.75, and the probability that he is a non-smoker is 0.25.

For convenience, one category (or event) is regarded as a 'success' and the other category (or failure of the event) as a 'failure'. The proportion π can be taken to refer to the proportion of successes in the population, and the proportion $(1 - \pi)$ as the proportion of failures. Thus, in the population of smokers above, the proportion of 'successes' is $\pi = 0.75$.

Now suppose a sample of size N is drawn from a population in which the proportion of successes is π. The proportion of successes in the sample is unlikely to be exactly equal to π, for just by chance the composition of the sample is unlikely to reflect exactly the composition of successes and failures in the population. Let us call the proportion of successes in the sample p. If repeated random samples of size N are taken, a number of sample proportions (p) will be generated which, as a result of sampling errors, will differ from one another and from the population proportion π. The reader will notice here the relationship between the population proportion π and the population mean μ, and the sample proportion p and the sample mean $\bar{X}$. Similarly, it can be shown that with repeated sampling the mean of the sample proportions p will tend to π (the population proportion), with a standard error given by $\sigma_p = \sqrt{[\pi(1 - \pi)/N]}$. This sampling distribution is called the binomial distribution.

Estimation procedures and tests of significance involving proportions are also quite common in medical statistics, and utilize the properties of the binomial distribution. However, provided N is large and π is not too close to 0 or 1, the binomial distribution approximates to the normal and the properties of the latter may be used in estimation or tests of significance.* Two examples are given below.

* If $\pi = 0.5$ the normal distribution can be used for values of N as low as 30. The further π is from 0.5 the larger should be the value of N to justify

EXAMPLE 6.1

A random sample of 100 adult females shows that 71 are smokers. Could this have been drawn from a population of adult females in which the proportion of smokers is 0·60?

Here $N = 100$, $\pi = 0·60$, $(1 - \pi) = 0·40$, $p = 0·71$.

The null hypothesis asserts that the sample has been drawn from a population with $\pi = 0·60$; the sample proportion differs from the population proportion only by chance. If repeated samples of 100 adult females are drawn from a population in which the proportion of smokers is 0·60, the sample proportions p will be approximately normally distributed around the population proportion π. The standard error of the distribution of the p's around π is given by

$$\sigma_p = \sqrt{[\pi(1 - \pi)/N]} = \sqrt{[0·60 \times 0·40/100]}$$

$$= 0·049$$

With $\sigma_p = 0·049$ the 95% confidence limits for p are given by

$$\pi \pm 1·96\sigma_p$$

$$= 0·60 \pm 1·96 \times 0·049$$

$$= 0·60 \pm 0·096$$

$$= 0·504 \text{ to } 0·696$$

The value of p obtained (0·71) falls outside these 95% confidence limits. If the hypothesis were true, the probability of obtaining a sample proportion p as different from the population proportion π as the one obtained, just due to chance, is very small (<0·05). We reject the null hypothesis at the 5% level of significance, and conclude that the sample could not have been drawn from a population in which the proportion of smokers is 0·60.

EXAMPLE 6.2

In a random sample of 150 medical practitioners, 33 are found

the use of the normal distribution as an approximation. It should also be noted that in substituting the normal for the binomial we are substituting a continuous for a discrete distribution.

to earn more than £10,000 per annum. Estimate with 95% confidence the proportion of all medical practitioners who earn more than £10,000 per annum.

In this example the problem is to estimate the population parameter π on the basis of the sample results. The proportion of medical practitioners in the sample who earn more than £10,000 per annum is $33/150 = 0.22$. Hence, $p = 0.22$ and $(1 - p) = 0.78$. In Chapters 3 and 4, it was explained how a sample mean $\bar{X}$ could be used to estimate the population mean (μ), by calculating the 95% confidence limits $\bar{X} \pm 1.96\sigma_{\bar{X}}$. The same procedure will be used here.

With $p = 0.22$, the 95% confidence limits for the estimate of π are given by $p \pm 1.96\sigma_p$. The standard error σ_p is calculated as $\sqrt{[\pi(1 - \pi)/N]}$. Since we do not know π, p is used instead (in the same way that, in previous examples, the sample standard deviation s was used instead of the unknown population standard deviation σ). This gives

$$\sigma_p = \sqrt{[p \times (1 - p)/N]} = \sqrt{[0.22 \times 0.78/150]}$$
$$= 0.034.$$

The 95% confidence interval for π is now calculated as

$$0.22 \pm 1.96 \times 0.034$$

$$= 0.22 \pm 0.067$$

$$= 0.153 \text{ to } 0.287$$

We can be 95% confident that between 15.3 and 28.7% of all medical practitioners earn more than £10,000 per annum.

The procedures used in both these examples are similar to those described in Chapters 3 and 4. Moreover, the techniques described in Chapter 4 for comparing two sample means $\bar{X}_1$ and $\bar{X}_2$ may be used to compare two sample proportions p_1 and p_2, on the null hypothesis that the two samples have been drawn from the same population or identical populations.

However, while the properties of the normal distribution can be used for tests of proportions involving large samples, they are inappropriate for small samples. For small samples different techniques based on the properties of the binomial distribution must be used.

6.4 Assumptions of sampling distributions

A fundamental assumption underlying tests of significance is that the sampling distribution of the statistic of interest corresponds to a particular hypothetical probability distribution. Many of the tests discussed in the previous chapters have rested on the assumption that the sampling distribution is normal. Other sampling distributions, such as the binomial distribution and Student's t distribution, have also been referred to. If the assumption concerning the sampling distribution is invalid, then the related tests of significance and the conclusions drawn from them are also invalid.

This important point is often overlooked. Thus it cannot be automatically assumed that the sampling distribution of the mean will be normal, even for quite large samples. If the parent population is normally distributed, the sampling distribution of the mean will also be normal, even for quite small samples. If the parent population is moderately skewed, the sampling distribution of means will tend to a normal distribution as the sample size increases, and may be assumed to be normal for large samples ($N > 30$). However, if the population is highly skewed, it cannot be assumed that the sampling distribution will be normal, even for large samples. It is therefore very important to examine the characteristics of a distribution before using any particular type of test of significance. For this purpose it is useful to draw a histogram or frequency polygon of a sample drawn from the population, since this gives an indication of how skewed the population might be.

While this subject will not be pursued here, it may be noted that various techniques are available for reducing the degree of skewness in a distribution. For example, while a variable X may be markedly skewed, it may be that $\log X$ is normal or nearly so. If $\log X$ is normally distributed it is referred to as a *log-normal distribution* and tests of significance may be used which are based on the characteristics of a log-normal distribution. Again, if a variable X is markedly skewed, it may be found that the transformed variable $1/X$ (the reciprocal transform) is normally or near-normally distributed. The use of transformations of this kind is quite common in medical statistics; many important variables, such as blood pressure and lipid levels, are found in practice to be markedly skewed, and skewness can be reduced by transforming the original data.

6.5 Sequential sampling

The tests of significance so far discussed have involved a 'fixed size' sampling procedure. Determination of sample size is one of the most important matters to be decided in designing an experiment. Techniques are available to aid the experimenter in deciding how large the sample size should be. Once the sample size has been determined, the experiment proceeds; when all the sample results have been collected, the sample data are analysed and a decision is made on the result of the experiment.

The main features of this type of sampling procedure are (1) the selection of a sample of a predetermined minimum size, and (2) a test of significance cannot be applied, and the experiment concluded, until all the sample results become available.

In medical research, it is sometimes inconvenient to conduct an experiment by means of a fixed-size sample. Suppose a new method of treatment of a particular disease is developed, and it is wished to compare this new method of treatment with an already established method. The new method of treatment is applied to a sample of patients, whilst for comparative purposes a suitably matched control group is treated by the established method. (Alternatively, for each matched pair entering the trial, one is given the new drug and the other a placebo.) If a fixed-size sampling procedure is used, a considerable period of time may elapse before sufficient patients are available to fill the sample 'quota'. It would be useful if each sample item could be tested as it became available, and the experiment terminated as soon as sufficient results had been obtained to make a decision on the efficacy of the new method of treatment. So, after a number of patients, or pairs of patients, had been tested it can be decided to (a) reject the null hypothesis that the new method of treatment is not significantly better than the established method, (b) accept the hypothesis, (c) continue the trial. Eventually a point will be reached where either decision (a) or (b) can be made, and the trial may be terminated.

Moreover, a fixed-size sample may be undesirable on ethical grounds. If one group of patients are being given a new drug, whilst a control group are receiving placebos, there may be good reasons for limiting, as far as possible, the number of patients involved in the experiment, and for terminating the experiment as soon as possible.

The type of sampling procedure called *sequential sampling* meets both requirements outlined above. In a sequential sampling scheme, sample items (for example, patients) may be tested as they become available, and the experiment terminated under the conditions stated above—analysis of the data may proceed continuously throughout the period of the experiment, instead of being dependent upon the completion of a fixed-size sample quota. In addition, it can be shown that, in general, the number of sample items required to reach a decision on the basis of a sequential sampling scheme is less than the number required for a fixed-size sample. This is obviously an important consideration in medical research experiments.

The statistical techniques involved in sequential sampling are a little complex and will not be discussed here, but a brief outline of the method will be given. Suppose it is wished to compare the effects of two different methods of treatment. As pairs of patients, suitably matched, become available, one of the pair receives Treatment A and the other Treatment B. For each patient, criteria are established for determining the success or failure of the treatment. For each pair of patients, four outcomes are possible; both Treatments a success, both Treatments a failure, Treatment A a success and Treatment B a failure, Treatment A a failure and Treatment B a success. For the purpose of the sequential test, the first two outcomes are described as 'tied pairs' and are discarded from the trial. Only the 'untied pairs' are used in the comparison of the two treatments. Now suppose we give a score of $+1$ to an outcome in which Treatment A is a success and B a failure, and a score of -1 to an outcome in which B is a success and A a failure. As the trial proceeds, a cumulative score is kept. It is evident that, if Treatment A is markedly superior to Treatment B, an increasing positive score will be cumulated, whilst an increasing negative score will cumulate in the reverse case. If there is no marked difference between A and B, then scores of $+1$ and -1 will occur in a random fashion, so that the total score will oscillate. These three possible outcomes are then used to make a decision about the relative efficiency of the two treatments.

The application of the sequential test makes use of a *sequential analysis chart*, and such a chart is shown in Example 6.3. In this example, the aim is to test the efficacy of Metoclopramide hydrochloride ('Maxolon') as a treatment for severe migraine; each patient takes Maxolon for a period of three months and a placebo for a period of three months (but not necessarily in that order). 'Untied pairs' in this trial occur when a definite preference is expressed *either* for Maxolon *or* for the placebo. The horizontal axis on the chart records the number of untied pairs included in the trial. The vertical axis records the cumulative score as the trial proceeds. As the results of each untied pair become available, the cumulative score is plotted against the number of untied pairs. In Example 6.3, the cumulative score is shown by the zigzag line.

It is now necessary to explain the meaning of the four 'boundary lines' marked on the chart. The trial may be terminated as soon as the score line reaches one of the boundary lines. If the score line crosses the upper boundary line, this is interpreted to mean that Maxolon is significantly better than the placebo. The opposite interpretation applies if the score line crosses the lower boundary line. Of course, the score line will not cross either boundary line unless a relatively high score has accumulated in favour of one or other of the treatments.

If, on the other hand, the score line crosses either of the

EXAMPLE 6.3

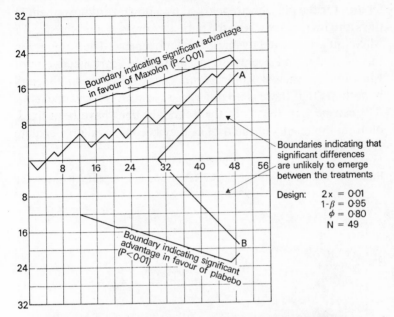

Sequential analysis graph showing therapeutic effect of 'Maxolon' (Metoclopramide) and of placebo, according to patient's preference. In each comparison the path is continued—one unit 'north-east' for preference for the first-named treatment and one unit 'south-east' for a preference for the second-named treatment. Redrawn from the *Practitioner*. Flavell Matts S. G. (1974), **212**, 887. Metoclopramide in the Treatment of Migraine. (By permission of the Author, Editor, and Publishers.)

boundary lines A or B, this is interpreted to mean that there appears to be no significant difference between the two methods of treatment. The score is not high enough in relation to the number of untied pairs tested to indicate a significant advantage of one treatment over the other.

The trial continues until the score line reaches one of the boundary lines, at which point a decision can be reached, at a predetermined level of significance, about the relative advantages of the two methods of treatment. In Example 6.3 the score line reached the upper boundary line after 48 untied pairs had been recorded. Cases where the patient showed a definite preference for the placebo are marked by a downward movement in the score line; cases where the patient expressed a preference for Maxolon are marked by an upward movement. The latter are in the majority, and eventually a cumulative score in favour of Maxolon is reached, sufficient to cause rejection of the null hypothesis that there is no difference between the treatments.

It can be seen that once the boundary lines have been fixed, plotting the results of the trial as they become available is quite

EXAMPLE 6.4

Effect of A.C.T.H. in facial palsy. Heavy line indicates seven successive pairs showing preference for A.C.T.H.

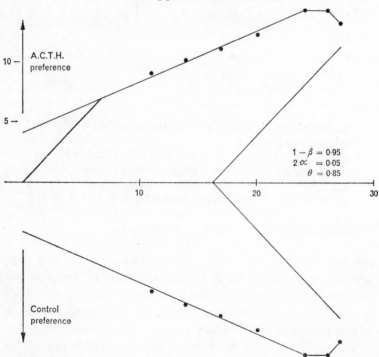

Reprinted from the *British Medical Journal*. Taverner D., Fearnley M. E., Kemble F., Miles D. W., and Peiris O. A. (1966), **1**, 391. Prevention of denervation in Bell's palsy. (By permission of the Authors, Editor, and Publishers.)

simple. The complexity of the technique lies in fixing the boundary lines for the particular experiment being conducted, and this will not be discussed here. For interpretative purposes, the boundary lines may be taken to correspond to confidence limits.

Another sequential sampling trial is shown in Example 6.4. Here the objective was to assess the effect of A.C.T.H. (adrenocorticotrophic hormone) in the treatment of Bell's palsy. As before, the trial concerned pairs of patients, one receiving A.C.T.H. and the other acting as a control. The axes and boundary lines of the chart are to be interpreted as for the previous example. The heavy line on the chart represents the cumulative score, and it will be seen to cross the upper boundary line following the outcome of the seventh untied pair. Each of the seven untied pairs was favourable to A.C.T.H. treatment, and it may be concluded from this analysis that there was a significant preference for this treatment.

If the score line had crossed either of the two 'middle' boundary lines, the trial would also have been terminated. In this case, it would be concluded that A.C.T.H. treatment offered no significant advantage in the treatment of Bell's palsy.

6.6   Analysis of variance

One of the most interesting and useful techniques in statistical analysis is the *analysis of variance*. In this section the basic concepts of analysis of variance will be explained. First, it is necessary to introduce another sampling distribution, called the *F* distribution.

It will be recalled that the measurement of variance was mentioned in Chapter 2, as the penultimate step in the calculation of the standard deviation. To calculate the variance of a sample of observations, the deviation of each sample item from the sample mean is squared, the squared deviations are added together and then divided by the total number of observations.*

---

* In statistical notation, this can be written $\Sigma(X - \bar{X})^2/N$. For small samples we divide by $(N - 1)$ rather than N, but this point may be overlooked here.

This is the variance. The standard deviation can then be calculated as the square root of the variance. Writing the sample standard deviation as s and the population standard deviation as σ, the sample variance and population variance may be written as s^2 and σ^2 respectively.

In Chapter 4, it was explained how to test the hypothesis that two samples have been drawn from the same population, by comparing the two sample means. If it can be shown that the difference between the two sample means is significant, then we may reject the null hypothesis that the two samples have been drawn from the same population or identical populations.

However, it is also possible to test the hypothesis that two samples have been drawn from the same population or identical populations by comparing the two sample variances. In comparing two sample means, it was noted that if the difference between them exceeded a certain critical value, the null hypothesis, that the two means are consistent with a common population mean μ could be rejected. Similarly, two sample variances may be compared, on the hypothesis that both variances are consistent with a certain common population variance. If the difference between the two variances exceeds a certain critical value, it may be concluded that the two samples could not have been drawn from the same population.

Actually, a test of the difference between two sample variances should logically precede a test of the difference between two sample means. If there is a significant difference between the two sample variances, then it is concluded that the two samples could not have been drawn from the same population; in this case it would be invalid to apply a test of the difference between the two sample means. In practice sample means are often compared without first comparing sample variances, and this can sometimes lead to erroneous conclusions.

The comparison of two sample variances involves what is called a *variance ratio test*. Suppose two samples are taken, and variances s_1^2 and s_2^2 are calculated, with $s_1^2 \geq$ (equal to or greater than) s_2^2. Now calculate

$$F = s_1^2/s_2^2$$

If the two sample variances are equal, then $s_1^2 = s_2^2$ and $F = 1$, and we may conclude that the two sample variances are estimates of the same population variance—the null hypothesis is accepted.

However, in the same way that the means of two samples drawn from the same population are likely to be different, just due to chance, the variances of these two samples are also likely to be different. In general, F will be greater than unity.* The greater the value of F, the greater the relative difference between the two sample variances, and the less likely it is that the two samples have been drawn from the same population. As for the χ^2 test, it can be established whether or not the value of F obtained is significant. If the value of F exceeds a certain critical value, it can be concluded that the two sample variances are significantly different; the null hypothesis, that the two samples have been drawn from the same population or identical populations, is rejected. As with other tests described, the F-test is strictly applicable only to samples drawn from a normal population, but may be used where the population does not differ markedly from the normal.

Having explained the F-distribution and variance ratio test, we are now in a position to discuss briefly the much more general area of *analysis of variance*. Paradoxically, despite its name and the use of the variance ratio test, analysis of variance is primarily concerned with comparing sample means. Unlike the techniques discussed in Chapter 4, however, analysis of variance is not confined to comparisons of two sample means.

Suppose a random sample of 100 observations is selected from a population and the sample mean and variance calculated. The sample mean and variance are unbiased estimates of the population mean and variance. Now suppose this sample is divided into four sub-samples, and the mean and variance calculated for each sub-sample. If the observations are randomly allocated amongst the sub-samples, each sub-sample may be regarded as a random sample from the same parent population; the means and variances of the four sub-samples should be

* The 'variance ratio' is calculated with the larger of the two sample variances as the numerator.

consistent with one another and with the population mean and variance.

Now let us suppose that the sample observations were not randomly allocated between the four sub-samples but were allocated to particular sub-samples or classes according to some criterion. For example, if the original sample of 100 referred to weights of males 21 years of age and over, we might classify these 100 weights into groups using a criterion of occupation. We may now ask—does weight vary with occupation? If there is no connection between weight and occupation, then each sub-sample may be regarded as before, as a random sample from the same population. The properties of the sub-samples should be consistent with one another. If, however, they are shown to be significantly different, it may be concluded that the sub-samples are not random samples drawn from a homogeneous parent population, but in fact have been drawn from different populations. In other words there is a connection between weight and occupation.

To answer this sort of problem, we set up the null hypothesis that *the variation in sample values is independent of the method of classification*. The null hypothesis is then tested by analysing the variation in values *within* each sub-sample and the variation in values *between* sub-samples. As a first step, the *total* variation in all the sample values is calculated; this is done by calculating the deviation of each sample value from the total sample mean, squaring the deviations and adding them together. This gives a measure of the total variation in all the sample values. This total variation can then be split into two components; the variation *within* sub-samples or classes, and the variation *between* classes. The methods by which this is done need not be explained here, but the general method of approach is illustrated in the simple example opposite.

Is there evidence of a difference between the three examiners with respect to marking? To answer this we set up the hypothesis that variations in marks are independent of the examiner concerned, and then test this hypothesis by an analysis of variance.

It will first be noted that there are variations in the marks

EXAMPLE 6.5

A random sample of 16 examination papers is taken and the results classified by examiner, as follows:

Examiner 1	Examiner 2	Examiner 3
74	74	76
72	77	78
71	73	79
74	75	78
74	76	76
		75

obtained within each group, which is to be expected. It may also be noted that there are variations in marks obtained *between* groups, as indicated by the fact that the *average marks obtained in each group are different*. The means of the three groups are 73, 75, and 77 marks respectively. The total variation in marks may be considered to consist of two components—the variation within groups and the variation between groups. The total variation may then be broken down to show (i) *the within sample variance* and (ii) the *between sample variance*.

We now reason as follows: If the null hypothesis were true, then each group could be regarded as a random sample from the same parent population—that is, the population of marks obtained by all candidates. Consequently, the variation in marks between samples should not be significantly different from the variation in marks within samples. If the null hypothesis is true, the within sample variance and the between sample variance are both independent estimates of the same population variance. If it can be shown that the within sample variance and the between sample variance are significantly different, by means of the variance ratio test, then doubt is cast on the hypothesis that the three samples have been drawn from the same parent population. We would conclude that marks obtained are not independent of examiner.

In this particular example, the between sample variance is 21·9, while the within sample variance is 2·3. It seems unlikely that

K

these two variances can be estimates of the same population variance. $F = 21 \cdot 9/2 \cdot 3 = 9 \cdot 5$, and this can be shown to be significant at the 1 % level. We reject the hypothesis that the three samples have been drawn from the same population. The between sample variance is too large in relation to the within sample variance. The variation in marks is not independent of the examiner.

In the simple example quoted above, the sample data are classified according to one criterion of classification—in this case, by examiner. Often, more than one criterion of classification is involved. In the example shown below two criteria are considered in analysing the variation in sample data—the birth rank of the infant, and maternal age. The null hypothesis is that differences in infant birth-weights are independent of birth rank or maternal age. The hypothesis is tested by estimating the share of the total variation in birth-weight which is attributable to differences in birth rank, and the share which is attributable to differences in maternal age, leaving a residual variation which is not attributable to either factor.

EXAMPLE 6.6

Two-factor analysis of variance. Variations in birth-weight analysed by birth rank and maternal age

Source of variation	D.F.	Sums of Squares	Mean Squares	Variance ratios	P values
Birth rank	3	56·81	18·94	14·80	$P < 0 \cdot 001$
Age	4	7·43	1·86	1·45	$P > 0 \cdot 20$
Birth rank × age	12	22·72	1·89	1·48	$0 \cdot 20 > P > 0 \cdot 05$
Residual	4,690	6,022·68	1·28		
Total	4,709	6,142·4			

Reprinted from the *British Journal of Preventive and Social Medicine*. Barron S. L., and Vessey M. P. (1966), **20**, 127. Birth weight of infants born to immigrant women. (By permission of the Authors, Editor, and Publishers.)

Under the column 'Sums of Squares' the total sum of squared deviations of birth-weights from the grand mean is shown as

6142·4. Using methods similar to those described in Example 6.5, 56·81 of this total variation is attributed to differences in birth rank, and 7·43 is attributed to differences in maternal age. If the effects of birth rank and age on birth-weight are strictly independent of one another, it is now only necessary to calculate the residual sum of squares, which is a measure of the variation in birth-weights due to other (random) effects. However, there may be *joint* effects in addition to the independent direct effects (compare this with the discussion of multiple regression in the previous chapter). This is the meaning of the 'birth rank × age' term in the table; it is an estimate of the joint or interaction effect of birth rank and age on the variation in birth-weights. Finally, the residual of 6022·68 is that part of the total variation in birth-weights not attributable to differences in birth rank or maternal age.*

The mean sum of squares or variance in each case is now calculated by dividing the total sum of squares by the number of degrees of freedom (which is derived from, but always somewhat less than, the number of observations). Now if the null hypothesis is true, the four estimates of variance calculated should be consistent. In particular each of the first three variance estimates should be consistent with the residual variance, which is in principle a measure of the variance in birth-weights due to other random effects. The variance ratio test is now applied to compare each 'attributed' variance with the residual variance. The F-ratios are shown in the second last column. The first one ($18·94/1·28 = 14·80$) is shown to be significant at the $0·1\%$ level ($P < 0·001$); if the null hypothesis were true, such a difference in variances would occur, due to chance, less than one in a thousand times. By convention the null hypothesis is rejected; birth-weights are not independent of birth rank.

In contrast, the F-ratios for age and the interaction of age and birth rank are not significant at the 5% level ($P > 0·05$); the

* For reasons which cannot be explained here, the component sums of squares in this example do not add up to the total sum of squares. In the more commonly used orthogonal analysis of variance, the residual sum of squares can be obtained by subtraction.

null hypothesis that birth-weight is independent of maternal age, and of the joint effect of maternal age and birth rank, is not rejected. Thus if birth-weights are classified by maternal age, we should not expect significant differences in mean birth-weights between age groups, once the effects of birth rank have been allowed for.

Analysis of variance can be extended to more than two criteria of classification. The technique may be seen to resemble multiple regression, in which the variation in one (dependent) variable can be broken down and attributed to a number of independent variables, which are the sources of the variation.

7

7.1 Vital statistics

A branch of statistics which is of particular interest in medical and social research is that concerned with the study of human population, often described as *demography*. Demographic studies involve *vital statistics* which we shall now consider.

Vital statistics are frequently used in medicine and so it is important that the more common measures should be outlined. They deal with statistics of death, birth, marriage, health, and disease. For the calculation of such measures the absolute numbers are transformed by prescribed formulae into rates or ratios. Thus we speak of birth rates, death rates, and so on. Absolute numbers would provide little information if it was wished to compare, for example, infant deaths between one area and another or one country and another, because the larger the population in an area then the larger the number of infant deaths is likely to be, although the relative figures may be identical.

Measures of mortality
The so-called *crude death rate* is defined as the number of deaths occurring during a calendar period per 1,000 of the average population during the same period, and is calculated as follows:

$$\frac{\text{Number of deaths occurring during a calendar period}}{\text{Average population during the same period}} \times 1,000$$

(Crude death rate, 1973; England & Wales—11·9; Ireland*— 11·2.)

---

* Excluding Northern Ireland. Reference to Ireland will in future exclude Northern Ireland.

If it is desired to compare the death rate in England and Wales with that in Ireland further calculation is necessary, and *standardized death rates* are estimated. It is obvious that death rates in any area will be influenced by the age and sex composition of the population. Elderly people have higher death rates than young people and males have higher death rates than females at most ages and from most causes. Hence, one would expect a population containing a high proportion of males and a high proportion of elderly people to have a higher crude death rate than a population with an excess of females and young persons. For this reason then the age and sex composition of the populations are important and will influence the crude death rate. To overcome these difficulties standardized death rates are estimated whereby adjustments are made for the age and sex compositions of the populations, which enable comparison to be made between these standardized rates. This allows a decision to be reached as to which of the populations has in fact got the higher death rate when age and sex is standardized, or held constant, in both populations. The calculation of standardized death rates is complex and will not be described here. They are, however, much more useful for purposes of comparison than crude death rates, whose uses are limited to analysis of short-term changes in mortality conditions. Standardized rates can be calculated to compare mortality conditions between different countries, different counties, and different occupations and social groups.

Death rates are often calculated for particular age groups and are called *age specific death rates*. An age specific death rate is defined as the number of deaths in a particular age group during a calendar period per 1,000 of the population of that age group during the same calendar period.

$$\frac{\text{Number of deaths in a particular age group during a calender period}}{\text{Population of that age group in the same calendar period}} \times 1{,}000$$

Age specific death rates can be calculated separately for each sex and in most countries the death rates for males for each age group are generally higher than for females in the same age group.

Another death rate or mortality rate of interest is the *infant mortality rate* and this rate is an index of medical and social standards in a community or in a country. It is defined as the number of deaths of infants under 1 year of age during a calendar period per 1,000 live births during the same period.

$$\frac{\text{Number of deaths of infants under 1 year of age during a calendar period}}{\text{Live births during the same period}} \times 1,000$$

(Infant mortality rate, 1973; England & Wales—16·9; Ireland—18·0.)

The infant mortality rate can be sub-divided into two further rates, the *neonatal mortality rate* and the *post-neonatal mortality rate*. The neonatal mortality rate is defined as the number of deaths of infants under 28 days during a calendar period per 1,000 live births during the same period.

$$\frac{\text{Number of deaths of infants under 28 days during a calendar period}}{\text{Live births during the same period}} \times 1,000$$

(Neonatal mortality rate, 1973; England & Wales—11·1; Ireland—12·7.)

The post-neonatal mortality rate is defined as the number of deaths of infants 28 days and over and under 1 year during a calendar period per 1,000 live births during the same period.

$$\frac{\text{Number of deaths of infants 28 days and over and under 1 year during a calender period}}{\text{Live births during the same period}} \times 1,000$$

(Post-neonatal mortality rate, 1973; England & Wales—5·8; Ireland—5·3.)

It is immediately obvious, as one would expect, that the sum of the neonatal and post-neonatal mortality rates provides the figure for the infant mortality rate. The reason for this sub-division of the infant mortality rate is because deaths in the early part of an infant's life are governed mainly by pre-natal influences, e.g. congenital malformation, immaturity, while deaths in the later part of the first year are more generally environmental in origin, e.g. pneumonia, bronchitis. It is important then to calculate different rates for these periods of an infant's life.

A *stillbirth rate* may also be calculated. This is defined as the number of stillbirths during a calendar period per 1,000 total (live and still) births during the same period.

$$\frac{\text{Number of stillbirths during a calendar period}}{\text{Total (live and still) births during the same period}} \times 1,000$$

(Stillbirth rate, 1973; England & Wales—11·6; Ireland—11·9.)

The *perinatal mortality rate* has received increased attention in recent years. It is defined as the number of stillbirths together with the number of deaths within the first seven days of life during a calendar period per 1,000 total (live and still) births in the same period.

$$\frac{\text{Number of stillbirths} + \text{deaths within the first 7 days of life during a calendar period}}{\text{Total (live and still) births during the same period}} \times 1,000$$

(Perinatal mortality rate, 1973; England & Wales—21·0; Ireland—22·9.)

There are several reasons for creating a perinatal mortality rate. Stillbirths and early neonatal deaths commonly have a similar aetiology, and the rate is regarded as an important index of the quality of obstetrical care. Further, since an infant who shows any sign of life is not regarded as being a stillbirth the perinatal mortality rate overcomes the difficulty of deciding whether or not an infant is stillborn.

A *maternal mortality rate* is defined as the deaths ascribed to puerperal causes during a calendar period per 1,000 total (live and still) births during the same period.

$$\frac{\text{Deaths ascribed to puerperal causes during a calendar period}}{\text{Total (live and still) births during the same period}} \times 1,000$$

(Maternal mortality rate, 1973; England & Wales—0·13; Ireland—0·13.)

The *case fatality (mortality) rate* is often of interest if it is desired to determine the proportion of patients with a particular disease or condition who die, e.g. in a diphtheria outbreak. It is defined as the number of deaths from a particular disease or condition as a percentage of the total numbers suffering from the disease or condition.

$$\frac{\text{Number of deaths from a particular disease or condition}}{\text{Total number suffering from the disease or condition}} \times 100$$

It has been explained how standardized death rates are used to compare mortality conditions between different populations by adjusting actual mortality rates (like the crude death rate) to account for differences in the age and sex composition of the populations being compared. In a similar way *standardized mortality ratios* can be computed and used for various forms of comparison, for instance, to examine mortality trends from a particular disease over a period of time.

TABLE 1. Standardized mortality ratios for
respiratory tuberculosis
(1968 = 100)

	1962	1967	1972
Males	178	108	66
Females	164	115	63

Source: Registrar General's Statistical Review of England and Wales, 1972, Part 1, H.M.S.O.

In simple terms the figures in Table 1 are computed as follows: the actual male and female mortality rates for this disease in 1968 are applied to the male and female populations of 1962, 1967, and 1972, to yield 'expected' deaths from respiratory tuberculosis in those years, i.e. the deaths which would have occurred if mortality rates in those years were identical to the 1968 rates. The ratio of *actual* deaths to 'expected' deaths in each year, multiplied by 100, is the standardized mortality rate (S.M.R.). The figures in the table tell us that actual deaths in 1962 were substantially

higher than 'expected', in other words that respiratory tuberculosis mortality rates in 1962 were higher than in 1968. Conversely,
in 1972 deaths were less than 'expected' (S.M.R. less than 100)
because mortality rates from respiratory tuberculosis have
declined since 1968. While the standardized mortality ratios for
respiratory tuberculosis have been declining the opposite trend
is seen for malignant neoplasm of trachea, bronchus, and lung.

TABLE 2

Leukaemia, aleukaemia	90
Vascular lesions of nervous system	110
Coronary disease, angina	118
General arteriosclerosis	125
Bronchitis	23
Nephritis and nephrosis	107
Suicide	176
Cirrhosis of liver	350
Malignant neoplasm of lung and bronchus	48
All causes	89
All males, all causes	100

Source: Registrar General's Decennial Supplement, England and
Wales, 1961, Occupational Mortality Tables, H.M.S.O.

Two other ways of using standardized mortality ratios are
illustrated in Tables 2 and 3. Table 2 shows standardized mortality ratios for *various conditions* for a *particular occupational
group* (medical practitioners). In this case, mortality rates for
these conditions for the total male population of England and
Wales aged 15–64 years are applied to male medical practitioners
aged 15–64. This yields the number of deaths expected if mortality rates amongst male medical practitioners aged 15–64 years
were identical to mortality rates in the whole male population
aged 15–64 years, for each condition. The ratio of actual to
expected deaths yields the standardized mortality ratio. From
this we see that mortality from suicide and cirrhosis of the liver,
for example, is above average (S.M.R. greater than 100), while
mortality from malignant neoplasm of the lung and bronchus is

much lower (S.M.R. less than 100). Mortality from all causes (89) is below average for the total male population aged 15–64 years.

TABLE 3

Farmers, farm managers, and market gardeners	63
Policemen	165
Electricians	101
Company directors	758
Bricklayers and tilesetters	83
Judges, barristers, etc., solicitors	93
Medical practitioners	118
Coal-miners (face workers)	144
Publicans	122
Athletes and sportsmen	107
University teachers	65
All males	100

Source: Registrar General's Decennial Supplement, England and Wales, 1961, Occupational Mortality Tables, H.M.S.O.

In Table 3, standardized mortality ratios for *various occupations* for a *particular disease*—in this case coronary disease and angina—are recorded. The interpretation, however, is similar. Thus, company directors have a markedly higher mortality (over $7\frac{1}{2}$ times) from coronary disease and angina than the general male population aged 15–64 years, while mortality amongst university teachers, and bricklayers and tilesetters is below average for the total male population aged 15–64 years.

While on the subject of mortality it is pertinent to include a short section on the accuracy of death certification. Studies of the accuracy of the certified cause of death have been conducted in five main ways. International comparisons of medical certificates of cause of death (Reid D. D. and Rose G. A., 1964, *Brit. med. J.*, **2**, 1437); clinical findings have been compared with those found at autopsy (Heasman M. A., 1962, *Proc. roy. Soc. Med.*, **55**, 733; Heasman M. A. and Lipworth L., 1966, *Accuracy of Certification of Cause of Death. Studies on Medical and Population Subjects*, No. 20, London, H.M.S.O.); evidence for the diagnosis on the certificate has been assessed by a questionnaire to the certifier (McKenzie A., 1956, *Brit. med. J.*, **2**, 204; Murphy T., 1967, *J. Irish med. Ass.*, **60**, 385); wording of the death certificate has been compared with the clinical diagnosis obtained from a study of clinical case notes (Alderson M. R. and Meade T. W., 1967, *Brit. J. prev. soc. Med.*, **21**, 22); and various causes of death have been related to the age of the certifying doctor (Bourke G. J. and Hall M. A., 1968, *J. Irish med. Ass.*, **61**, 115). All of these studies using different approaches have demonstrated considerable inaccuracies in certification and shown it to be subject to various errors. There are three important reasons why accurate statistics of mortality are required; firstly, mortality data are frequently used to identify associated factors, e.g. occupation; secondly, mortality data are necessary to plan health services and later to evaluate these services, e.g. screening for cervical cancer; and finally, such data are of importance in research studies of an epidemiological type. For these reasons then the medical profession must endeavour to determine accurately the condition from which a patient has died. It is not possible here to enter into a discussion of methods of improving accuracy of death certification but increasing autopsy rates will help considerably, although it should be emphasized that autopsies are not a complete answer. There is, among other things, a great need for education of medical graduates and undergraduates in the correct method of death certification and of the importance of determining the true cause of death.

Measures of fertility

The *birth rate*, or *crude birth rate*, is defined as the number of live births occurring during a calendar period per 1,000 of the average population during the same period.

$$\frac{\text{Number of live births occurring during a calendar period}}{\text{Average population during the same period}} \times 1,000$$

(Birth rate, 1973; England & Wales—13·7; Ireland—22·5.)

The crude birth rate, like the crude death rate, is of limited value since it depends upon the age and sex composition of the population. Specifically the rate is influenced by the number of women of child-bearing age in that population, and because it relates to the total population it does not necessarily indicate the relative fertility of that population. For this reason a *general fertility rate* is calculated. This is defined as the number of live births occurring during a calendar period per 1,000 women of child-bearing age in the population during the same period of time.

Since the general fertility rate is based only upon the number of women of child-bearing age in the population (in Ireland this is taken as the age range 15–49), it is clearly a better measure of fertility than the crude birth rate. However, the general fertility rate is also limited because it does not take into account the age-distribution of women of child-bearing age within the population. For this reason *age-specific fertility rates* (similar to age-specific mortality rates) are calculated, from which a further measure called the *total fertility rate* is calculated. The total fertility rate represents an estimate of the average number of children born to a woman throughout her child-bearing period, subject to prevailing age-specific fertility rates. Thus a total fertility rate of 3,700 per 1,000 implies that, on average, 1,000 women would be expected to bear a total of 3,700 children throughout their child-bearing age span. The calculation of this rate is an example of the use of cohort analysis which is discussed in the following section.

The concept of the total fertility rate is closely related to analysis of population trend. In analysis of population trends, the important factor to be determined is whether or not the female population is replacing itself from one generation to the next, for in the long run this determines the trend in total population. For this purpose *gross* and *net reproduction rates* are calculated. The gross reproduction rate is similar to the total fertility rate, except that it refers to *female* births only; thus if it happened that males and females were born in equal numbers, a total fertility rate of 3,700 per 1,000 would give rise to a gross reproduction rate of 1,850 per 1,000. The net reproduction rate is derived from, and is slightly less than, the gross rate—it takes account of mortality conditions as they affect women throughout the child-bearing span. In summary, the net rate measures the average number of female children born to a woman during her child-bearing life, subject to prevailing specific fertility and specific mortality rates.

Measures of Morbidity
Morbidity, which is ill-health or sickness, may cause diffi-culties in measurement. Death is an event which occurs at one point in time while sickness may last for a period of time, may recur, and may present with different degrees of severity. In addition, a person may have more than one illness. It is not intended to enter into any detail about morbidity statistics, but before this section on vital statistics is concluded there are two rates connected with morbidity, as distinct from mortality, which are in common use and must be explained. These two rates are the *incidence rate* and the *prevalence rate* and they are often con-fused. An incidence rate is defined as the number of cases of a particular disease or condition *commencing* during a specified time per 100 of the average population during the same period of time.

$$\frac{\text{Number of cases of a particular disease or}}{\text{condition } \textit{commencing} \text{ during a specified time}} \times 100$$
$$\frac{}{\text{Average population during the same period of time}} \times 100$$

The prevalence rate which is commonly used is known as the *point prevalence rate*. The point prevalence rate is defined as the number of cases of a particular disease or condition *existing in* a population at a specified time per 100 of the population at that time.

$$\frac{\text{Number of cases of a particular disease or}}{\text{condition } \textit{existing in} \text{ a population at a specified time}} \times 100$$
$$\frac{}{\text{Population at that time}} \times 100$$

Incidence and prevalence rates are usually expressed as a percentage although other multiplying factors may be used. This, of course, presents no difficulty provided it is stated clearly what the multiplying factor is. Incidence is concerned with the number of *new* cases of a disease or condition occurring, while prevalence is concerned with the *total number* of cases in a population.

7.2 Life tables and cohort analysis

In the previous section, a number of measures of mortality were described. One important measure of mortality which was not covered is the *mean expectation of life at birth*. The calculation of life expectancy involves what are called *life tables*, and is a special example of a form of statistical analysis termed *cohort analysis*. The general characteristics of cohort analysis, and in particular its use in constructing life tables, will now be explained.

The disadvantages of the crude death rate as a measure of comparative mortality have already been pointed out. A comparison of crude death rates between countries A and B, or within the same country at different periods of time, may not be very meaningful because of differences in the age and sex compositions of the two populations. Ideally, we should like to ask— what would the crude death rates be if the two countries had identical populations? Another way of expressing this is to ask— what is the average expectation of life of an individual in each country? It is to answer this question that life tables are constructed.

The construction of life tables will now be explained with reference to Table 4. Suppose we postulate a *cohort* of 100,000

TABLE 4. Irish life table 1960–62—males

Age x	l_x	d_x	L_x	T_x	$\overset{\circ}{e}_x$	Age x
0	100,000	3,131	97,248	6,813,226	68·13	0
1	96,869	214	96,762	6,715,978	69·33	1
2	96,655	123	96,594	6,619,216	68·48	2
3	96,532	82	96,491	6,522,622	67·57	3
4	96,450	68	96,416	6,426,131	66·63	4
5	96,382					

Source: *Irish Statistical Bulletin*, Volume XL, No. 2, June 1965, p. 88. (Table abbreviated), Government Publication.

male births in a particular year. A number of the cohort will die during the first year of life (infant mortality). In Ireland, the number who die could be estimated by means of the current infant mortality rate. In the period 1960–62, the average male infant mortality rate for Ireland was 31·31 per 1,000, so that out of 100,000 male births the 'expected' number of deaths can be estimated as 3,131. Thus, of the original cohort 96,869 may be expected to survive to age 1. These figures are shown in the columns headed l_x and d_x in the table.

How many of our hypothetical cohort will survive to age 2? This can be estimated by using the actual current (1960–62) specific mortality rates for Ireland for the age group 1 and under 2 years of age. Thus, it is estimated that 214 of the cohort will die between the ages of 1 and 2, leaving 96,655 to survive until age 2.

The general procedure will now be clear. At each age, the cohort is subjected to the specific mortality rates for that age group. Eventually, of course, the cohort will 'die off'. The number who die at each age is determined by the specific mortality rates, and these are usually based on the average mortality rates for the most recent period for which accurate statistics are available.

Consider now the column headed L_x. The figures in this column measure the estimated total number of years lived by the cohort at each age. To explain this, suppose the whole cohort had survived to age 1 (the infant mortality rate was zero). In this case, the total number of years lived by the cohort, between birth and age 1, would be 100,000—each member of the cohort would have lived for 1 year.

However, it is estimated that only 96,869 of the cohort live for a year, while 3,131 live for only part of a year. Thus, the total number of years lived by the cohort is 96,869 plus some fraction of 3,131. The precise method of calculation will not be explained here*—in summary, it is estimated that the total number of years lived by the cohort, between the ages of 0 and 1, is 97,248.

---

* The simplest assumption would be that those who die live on average six months each, so that the 3,131 of the cohort who die before reaching age 1 would live for a total of $3,131/2 = 1,565·5$ years. This assumption is made

Similarly, the total number of years lived by the cohort between the age of 1 and 2 is 96,655 (the number of years lived by the survivors to age 2) plus some fraction of 214 (those who die before reaching the age of 2). This is estimated to be 96,762. The interpretation of the L_x column should now be clear.

Turning now to the T_x column, the first figure in this column is the total number of years lived by the cohort at all ages—in fact, the sum of *all* the figures in the L_x column. Thus, the life span of all the members of the cohort is estimated to account for a total of 6,813,226 years. Since we started off with 100,000 persons in the cohort, the average number of years lived by the cohort is $6,813,226 \div 100,000 = 68 \cdot 13$ years. This average, recorded in the last column of the table, is the mean expectation of life at birth of an Irish male. It tells us how many years an Irish male may be expected to live—or, alternatively, the average age of an Irish male at death—subject to certain specific mortality conditions.

The other entries in columns T_x and $\mathring{e}_x$ are also of interest. For example, the second figure in the T_x column measures the total number of years lived by the cohort from the age of 1 onwards; the second figure (69·33) in the $\mathring{e}_x$ column is derived from this, and measures the *mean expectation of life at age 1*. That is, a male who has survived to age 1 may expect on average to live a further 69·33 years. Thus, the figures in the $\mathring{e}_x$ column measure the average expectation of life at all ages.

There are many other features of life tables which could be discussed, but sufficient has been explained to demonstrate their importance in analysis of mortality. Life tables can be constructed for different populations and comparisons made on the basis of life expectancy. Separate tables can be constructed for males and females, for different social groups, and for different occupations. Comparisons can be made which are independent of the effects of age and sex composition; and the mean expectation of life is a useful and simple concept to understand.

The use of cohort analysis was also referred to in discussing the

for all age groups *except* the age group 0 to 1, since most deaths in this group occur in the first months of life.

measurement of fertility, in particular the calculation of the total fertility rate and related measures. Here we start with a cohort of women of child-bearing age and subject the cohort to specific fertility rates as the cohort passes through each age group. From this, the total number of children born to the cohort can be estimated, giving rise to the total fertility rate. Like the mean expectation of life, this is an hypothetical measure and depends upon the assumption of certain specific fertility rates.

As explained, the advantage of cohort analysis is that it eliminates the effects of variable factors such as the age and sex composition of a population, which may obscure underlying trends in, for example, mortality and fertility.

A more general application of cohort analysis is shown in Example 7.1. Here the aim is to compare the age-specific mortality experience from cancer of the bladder of successive generations of women aged 50–84.

The parallel diagonal lines in the table are boundaries between successive cohorts. Thus, consider the value 0·286, which is the eighth figure from the left in the first row of the table. This indicates that the mortality rate per 1,000 for the age group 80–84 (noted in the far left column) was 0·286 in the period 1946–50 (as noted in the bottom row). Simple calculation tells us that women aged 80–84 in 1946–50 must have been born in the period around 1865 (noted in the top row of the table); this is the cohort whose mortality experience is recorded. Moving downwards to the left along the tranche formed by the diagonal lines, we note that in the period 1941–45, when members of the cohort were aged 75–79 years, the age-specific mortality rate was 0·223 per 1,000 (or 223 per million). Continuing, age-specific mortality for this cohort was 154 per million at age 70–74, 94 per million at age 65–69, and so on down to 20 per million at age 50–54. Reading *up* the tranche, we note that age-specific mortality increases with age.

The other tranches can be similarly interpreted, as showing the mortality experience of successive cohorts of women aged 50–84, each cohort being distinguished by date of birth. Since records of mortality from 1911–15 to 1966–70 were employed in the

EXAMPLE 7.1

Mortality (per 1,000) from cancer of the bladder 1911–70 in England and Wales, women aged 50–84 years, with median year of birth indicated on the diagonals

Age	Year of birth												Year of birth—contd.
	1830	1835	1840	1845	1850	1855	1860	1865	1870	1875	1880	1885	
80–84	0·135	0·137	0·211	0·184	0·218	0·221	0·224	0·286	0·349	0·364	0·349	0·397	
75–79	0·153	0·131	0·156	0·188	0·186	0·201	0·223	0·239	0·266	0·267	0·267	0·276	1890
70–74	0·116	0·117	0·116	0·135	0·150	0·154	0·146	0·174	0·169	0·174	0·172	0·179	1895
65–69	0·078	0·080	0·098	0·106	0·094	0·106	0·107	0·120	0·111	0·119	0·108	0·114	1900
60–64	0·056	0·058	0·067	0·061	0·059	0·068	0·075	0·074	0·065	0·068	0·066	0·067	1905
55–59	0·035	0·034	0·038	0·036	0·037	0·040	0·041	0·040	0·043	0·039	0·041	0·041	1910
50–54	0·019	0·020	0·022	0·022	0·018	0·023	0·027	0·026	0·025	0·021	0·023	0·020	1915
	1911 –15	1916 –20	1921 –25	1926 –30	1931 –35	1936 –40	1941 –45	1946 –50	1951 –55	1956 –60	1961 –65	1966 –70	

Year of death

Reprinted from the *British Journal of Preventive and Social Medicine*. Armstrong B., and Doll R. (1974), **28**, 233. Bladder cancer mortality in England and Wales in relation to cigarette smoking and saccharin consumption. (By permission of the Authors, Editor, and Publishers.)

study, the earliest cohort is that for women born around 1830. This tranche has only one entry (the top left-hand figure in the table) as mortality in age groups above 84 was not considered. Similarly the latest cohort is for 1915, since later cohorts would be aged less than 50 in the period 1966–70. Reading across the *rows* of the table enables us to compare the mortality experience of different cohorts at similar ages. The reader should, however, consult the reference cited for detailed analysis of the data.

7.3 Computers and medical research

It is appropriate to complete this book by a brief discussion of the role of the modern electronic computer in medical and social research. In recent years computers have proved an invaluable aid to many aspects of medical and social research work. It is no exaggeration to state that, without the computer, certain studies would be impossible to initiate. Although, in principle, the functions performed by the computer can be performed 'manually', in practice the immense amount of sorting and analysis which is involved in many studies would not be feasible without the aid of a computer.

In simplest terms a computer can be defined as a calculating machine able to perform a wide variety of basic functions very rapidly. Although a computer is capable of carrying out extremely complex operations, it can only operate in the way it has been instructed by the user.

The series of related instructions required to deal with a particular problem or activity (like sorting data into tables, or calculating and comparing the means of two samples) form a *programme*, which provides a step by step course for the computer to follow. Of course, if a problem cannot be defined and formulated in detail, then it is not possible to programme it for solution by the computer. Quite often it is the definition of the problem that creates the most difficulty.

Special programmes are required to control the activities of the computer system itself and these are given the general name of 'system software'. The actual physical pieces of equipment making up the computer form the 'hardware'. The hardware consists of a number of units, such as:

The central processor which provides central control over the functioning of the entire system and interprets the instructions of any programme

The arithmetic unit which performs all the arithmetic and logical functions of the computer, and works on the data which are held in the memory unit

The memory storage unit which holds the programmes which are to be used, the actual data and the systems software in such a manner that this can be made available to the central processor during the execution of the programme

The input/output control unit which provides the means by which programmes and data can enter the system, and results leave it. Connected to this control unit are 'peripherals' such as paper tape readers, card readers, line printers and magnetic tape units.

Although the cost of computer time per hour may appear very high, when considered in light of the amount of work performed in that time the cost becomes far more reasonable—especially when sophisticated software techniques are used enabling numerous programmes to be run together. Most modern computers perform individual operations in a few millionths of a second (microseconds), and it is common for powerful computers to be able to carry out more than a million additions in a second.

Computer applications fall into a number of different types or classes, and computer systems vary in their design according to the type of application required. For example, some computers may be designed for fairly routine data processing—such as invoicing or the preparation of payrolls—while others may be designed for high-speed scientific calculations.

For medical or social work, the computer applications which are mainly of interest are data processing and the solution of statistical problems or statistical calculations. For example, suppose it is decided to conduct a large-scale retrospective survey on coronary heart disease. The first step will be to prepare carefully a list of all the data required (such as age, sex, diagnosis, blood pressure, weight, smoking experience, occupation), as well as coding instructions and code reference numbers, which will be explained in a moment. This list of data requirements and instructions, which is sometimes called a 'protocol', is worth drafting very carefully, preferably in conjunction with a statistician and/or the person responsible for the computer application. A carelessly prepared protocol can lead to awkward problems at a later stage of the project.

The next step is to collect the data required, and this will normally entail a questionnaire or record sheet for each person included in the survey. The design of the questionnaire or record sheet is also an important preparatory stage of the study, and this should also be done in conjunction with the statistician and/or person in charge of the computer application. It is important that the design of the questionnaire conforms to the instructions set out in the protocol.

When the record sheets are completed—or as they become available—the data are then converted into a form suitable for acceptance by the computer. Usually, punch cards are used. The data from each record sheet are punched on to a card, which can be 'read' by the computer via the input/output control unit. This is the purpose of the coding instructions which are set out in the protocol. For example, the following information may be collected in the record sheet (Fig. 7.1).

Each person in the survey is given a number, for purposes of identification. If the number of persons in the survey runs into four figures, then four columns will be required on the punch card. Thus, if the survey number is 259, the first card column will be left blank or punched 0, while positions 2, 5 and 9 will be punched in columns 2, 3 and 4 respectively.

The coding instructions for sex are that 1 will be punched for a male, and 2 for a female. Thus, if the patient is male, the number 1 will be ringed, and this will be punched in column 5 of the card.

The treatment of variables such as age and weight depend on how precise we wish this information to be. In the example, age groups have been used; if the patient is, say, 34 years of age the code number 3 is ringed and this will be punched in column 6.

	Code Number	Columns
Survey Number	0259	1 – 4
Sex ①. Male	1	5
2. Female		
Age 1. Under 20 years	3	6
2. 20–29 years		
③. 30–39 years		
4. 40–49 years		
5. 50 years and over		
Weights (lbs.) *153*	153	7 – 9

FIG. 7.1

However, we may wish the data on weight to be expressed to the nearest pound, in which case the actual weight of the patient is recorded (for instance 153 lb). Three columns will be required for this on the punch card.

In order that the data can be transferred on to punch cards with the minimum error and maximum efficiency, it is obviously important that the coding instructions be carefully established and that the lay-out of the record sheet should facilitate punching as far as possible. In the example shown, it is only necessary for the punch card operator to read down the column headed 'code number'. It would be possible to punch the data from the left-hand column, where numbers are ringed or written in, but most record sheets contain a considerable amount of data, and reading through the data to find the appropriate number to punch can sometimes be confusing and lead to mistakes; it also takes far longer than reading down a single column of numbers. Usually the data are first compiled by ringing or writing-in the appropriate numbers under 'sex', 'age', and so on; it is then advisable to fill up the column headed 'code number', from which the card operator will transfer the data on to the punch cards. Where this has not been done, record sheets are often so confusing that they have to be 're-processed' before punching can begin, and this is time-consuming and irritating to all concerned.

The typical punch card has 80 columns (see Fig. 7.2) and if there are more than 80 columns to be used a second card will be required for each person. If more than one card is required, it is often useful to repeat certain pieces of information, such as the survey number and patient's sex and age, on the second and subsequent decks of cards.

As soon as the punch cards are completed and programmes prepared,* the data can be fed into the computer for processing and analysis. In a survey, it is common to prepare a large number of tables, of frequency distributions, bi-variate classifications and so on. For example, we may wish to classify male and female patients by age. Given the instructions, the computer will sort the cards and print out the required table. The preparation of tables of this kind is a routine computer application.

The computer may also be used for tests of significance, fitting regression equations and similar statistical and mathematical operations. It need hardly be stressed that, in a large-scale survey, the preparation of numerous tables and statistical calculations would be an extremely arduous task without the assistance of a computer. Even quite 'small' problems, such as fitting a regression equation for 30 pairs of observations, involves a considerable amount of work. The computer is an indispensable aid in modern research methods.

Most readers will be familiar with the term *medical record linkage* which as its name suggests is a means of bringing together selected data from medical records. Prior to the introduction of computers national and area statistics generally related to single events, since the task of linking together several events for individuals was one of great magnitude, e.g. diagnoses in recurrent admissions to different hospitals. When computers were introduced such linking of data became feasible. It was now possible to put medical records to better use and to store collected information on cards or tape in a small space. Further, this information could be retrieved more quickly than before, cumulative files for

---

* The programme may be specially written for a particular problem. However, a large and growing number of 'standard' programmes are now available to tackle many types of problems.

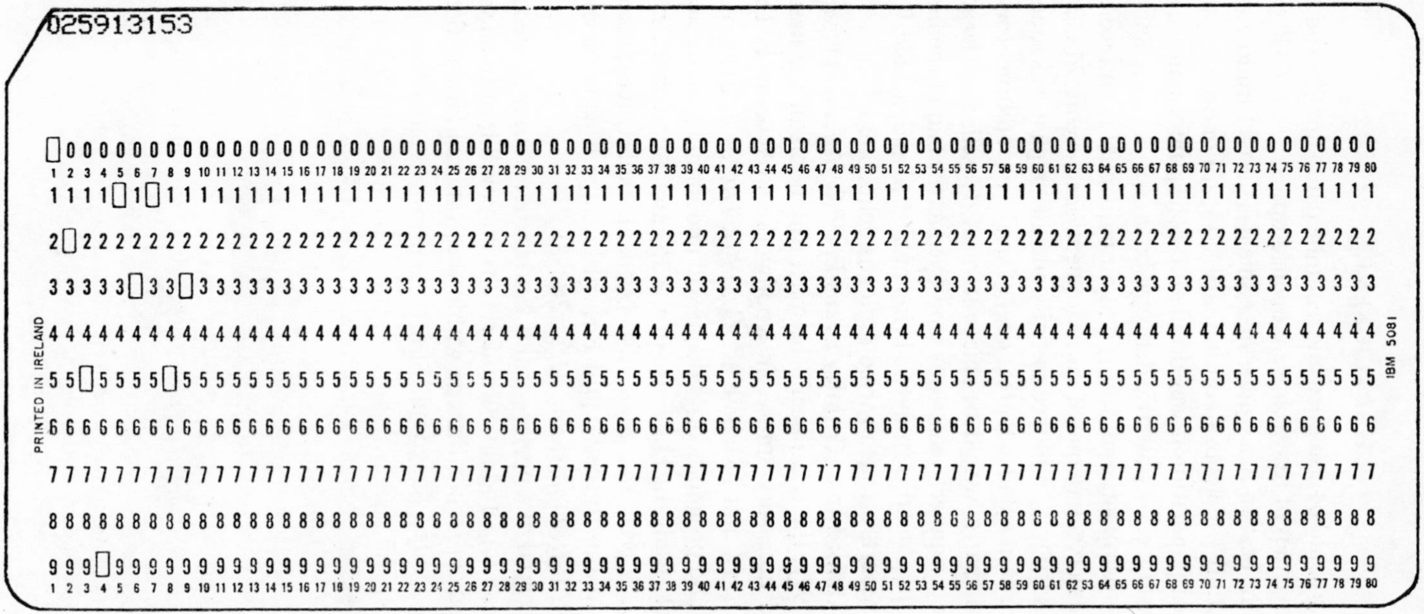

Fig. 7.2
(By courtesy of IBM Ireland Limited)

individuals could be compiled and assembled into family groups, and new avenues of research were opened up.

One of the best known studies in this field is the Oxford Record Linkage Study which began on January 1, 1962. For each person in a defined population it was decided to collect information, in the first instance, on obstetric delivery, birth, periods of hospital in-patient treatment, and death; and an individual is entered in the study as a result of one of the aforementioned events. Manual record linkage was employed initially and although it was found to be efficient, it entailed a great deal of work; in addition, it was considered that it would be uneconomical if used on a larger scale, so a computer system was employed at the end of the first year. Results from this study are being published and include, for example, reports on such varied topics as deliberate self-poisoning in the Oxford area (Grimley Evans J., 1967, *Brit. J. prev. soc. Med.*, **21**, 97); the relationship between carcinoma of the nasal cavity and accessory sinuses in woodworkers (Acheson E. D., Hadfield E. H. and Macbeth R. G., 1967, *Lancet*, **1**, 311); the incidence and prognosis of undiagnosed abdominal pain treated in hospital (Rang E. H., Fairbairn A. S. and Acheson E. D., 1970, *Brit. J. prev. soc. Med.*, **24**, 47); and sudden unexpected deaths in infants in the Oxford Record Linkage Area (Fedrick, Jean, 1974, *Brit. J. prev. soc. Med.*, **28**, 93).

The potential of a project of this kind is enormous in terms of medical research, and favourable results may well lead to a system of medical record linkage within the National Health Service in the United Kingdom.

Suggestions for Further Reading

There are many books on statistics, at varying levels of complexity. Most of the books listed below are aimed primarily at readers with an interest in medicine and allied areas of study. This interest is reflected both in the examples chosen and in the relative emphasis given to different applications and concepts of statistical inference.

For the reader who seeks a good grasp of the basic concepts of statistical inference and their application to medical research, the following are recommended:

Armitage P., *Statistical Methods in Medical Research* (Blackwell Scientific Publications, Oxford, 1971)
Remington R. D. and Schork M. A., *Statistics with Application to the Biological and Health Sciences* (Prentice-Hall, Englewood Cliffs, 1970)

Less comprehensive, but nevertheless also useful are:

Bahn A. K., *Basic Medical Statistics* (Grune & Stratton, 1972)
Moroney M. J., *Facts from Figures* (Pelican, 1962)
Hill A. Bradford, *Principles of Medical Statistics*, 9th edition (The Lancet, London, 1971)
Goldstein A., *Biostatistics—an introductory text* (Macmillan, New York, 1962)
Mainland D., *Elementary Medical Statistics* (W. B. Saunders Philadelphia, 1963)

An excellent book on the subject of vital statistics is:

Benjamin B., *Health and Vital Statistics* (Allen & Unwin, 1968)

(For up-to-date statistics and commentary, the *United Nations Demographic Yearbook* is a very good source.)

Index

Testing hypotheses 48, 49–50, 70–2

Tests of significance (*see* Significance)

Time series 6

Treatment group 66

Variable 2

continuous 3
dependent 101
discrete 3
independent 101
Variance 39, 135–7
  analysis of 135–42
  between sample 139
  ratio test 136–7
  within sample 139
Vital statistics 143–53